Professionalism and Ethics in Medicine

Laura Weiss Roberts • Daryn Reicherter
Editors

Professionalism and Ethics in Medicine

A Study Guide for Physicians and Physicians-in-Training

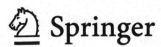 Springer

Editors
Laura Weiss Roberts, MD, MA
Department of Psychiatry
and Behavioral Sciences
Stanford University School of Medicine
Stanford, CA, USA

Daryn Reicherter, MD
Department of Psychiatry
and Behavioral Sciences
Stanford University School of Medicine
Stanford, CA, USA

ISBN 978-1-4939-1685-6   ISBN 978-1-4939-1686-3 (eBook)
DOI 10.1007/978-1-4939-1686-3
Springer New York Heidelberg Dordrecht London

Library of Congress Control Number: 2014955727

Printed on acid-free paper

Springer is part of Springer Science+Business Media (www.springer.com)

*For Anne and Leonard Weisskopf, nurse
and physician, my mother and late father*

– LWR

*For Heidi, Ethan, and Amelia,
the inspiration for everything I do*

– DR

Foreword

> A hero is someone who understands the responsibility that comes with his freedom.
>
> Bob Dylan

Physicians are entrusted with caring for patients and serving the health of the public. In this work, physicians encounter hard questions: questions that test their assumptions about what is "right" and "wrong," questions that test the professional roles of the doctor in the modern world, and questions that test their human heart. When may a woman refuse life-prolonging treatment? When may a trainee accept a gift from a patient? When may a mother decline to have her child immunized? When should a doctor confront a colleague with concerns about impairment, misconduct, or harassment? When must a physician report suspected abuse or dangerousness? *Professionalism and Ethics in Medicine: A Study Guide for Physicians and Physicians-in-Training* is a down-to-earth reference to help clarify and resolve such complex issues encountered across the field medicine.

This text provides a framework for learning that is informed by the emerging understanding of medical professionalism in a culturally diverse and technologically advancing world. The framework is also informed by the traditions of western bioethics and the law. With this foundation, readers of this text are provided with vignettes, cases, and prompts that derive from real-life clinical practice, research, and educational settings. Vignettes are found in each chapter of the first section of the book; they are rich and complex and they are intended to stimulate self-reflection and inspire discussion. The later sections of the book are entirely devoted to cases and prompts in the form of questions and answers, with Part II providing narrative explanations. The vignettes, cases, and prompts serve to reinforce understanding of both evolving and enduring aspects of professionalism and ethics in present-day medicine.

This book was built through the work of many physicians and physicians-in-training who contributed case material from many perspectives: diverse disciplines of medicine; diverse patient populations; diverse domains of medical practice, science, and training; and diverse roles and settings for care. Readers of this *Study Guide* will work through issues encountered by surgeons and pediatricians, psychiatrists and internists, by military doctors, by academic faculty, by rural and urban physicians, by immigrant physicians, by medical students and residents, and others.

The *Study Guide* is meant to broadly represent medicine, but it does not claim to be comprehensive, and given rapid changes in society, it is certainly not timeless. This book can inform but never substitute for the mature judgment of a thoughtful physician. Nevertheless, ethics principles, guidelines for culturally astute care, legal precedents, and ideals of professionalism come to life through the case material highlighted throughout the text. The *Study Guide* should help practitioners and trainees to prepare for examinations that assess professionalism, ethics, and related topics. It is our hope that the reader will translate the insights from this book to their own work – that the *Study Guide* will help our readers to apply the principles, guidelines, precedents, and ideals to their activities and roles, and that their skill in this will expand and adapt as their professional lives unfold.

Stanford, CA, USA   Laura Weiss Roberts
                                                        Daryn Reicherter

Preface

When the Middle Path Intersects the Way of the Cross

In an effort to provide culturally appropriate care for the Khmer community in San Jose, California, my clinic was in discussion with the Buddhist monks at the local temple about partnership. Many of the Khmer refugee population who relocated to San Jose lived in a low-income area and remained very isolated. Many Khmer refugees did not receive adequate healthcare or mental health treatment because of barriers of language and culture, as well as financial, social, and transportation limits. And many did not have healthcare because they just did not know how to access it.

The neighborhood served by our clinic was a true cultural "melting pot" with as much diversity as one can imagine. Immigrants from El Salvador shared playgrounds with children from Vietnam. Shop signs in the same strip mall were posted in Spanish, Vietnamese, Chinese, Korean, Khmer, and even English. Our clinic, by definition, had to be culturally sensitive and culturally competent in order to conduct its work each day.

The temple was in the midst of the Khmer community and in the middle of Silicon Valley, an enclave of poverty in the shadow of billion-dollar high-tech companies like Google, Yahoo, and Facebook.

We wanted to discuss with the monks ways that we could create greater connection to healthcare through the temple. Patient confidentiality, boundary issues, and clear roles in healthcare were just some of the ethical and professional concerns we thought. For the Khmer, the temple is the center of the community, and the monk is the center of the temple. It is certainly not the doctor and definitely not white, English-speaking doctors who play a leadership role for their community. Beginning partnership with the Khmer monks catalyzed my education in the real issues of cultural sensitivity and opened a dialogue that explored the limits of Western professionalism and medical ethics in a multicultural context.

We met in a house-turned-temple in a neighborhood known for crime, with bars on the windows and broken glass in the street. This temple maintained the respect of the community, although it lacked the glory of Khmer architecture seen in Cambodia. The Khmer social worker from my clinic genuflected when the monks came in and bowed her head, forehead to the floor. We sat cross-legged, in a converted garage filled with incense, under a mural of the Banyan Tree with a giant golden Buddha covered in brightly-colored lights behind. The abbot spoke for the monks, his English far better than my Khmer. Despite many years as a healthcare provider for Khmer speakers and some professional travel in Cambodia, I only knew basic greetings.

Choum Reap sour, I greeted with an unconvincing accent, with my hands clasped in the traditional *sampeah* greeting. Very formal.

The monks were disarmed by my attempt at cultural appropriateness and smiled.

Sok sabay, the abbot returned. It means "happy, healthy." Very informal. And the monks laughed.

The brilliant conversation that followed was full of enthusiasm and frustration. It was clear that we all shared a common goal of supporting the Khmer community in accessing health and mental healthcare. But some basic ethical and professional questions were tested by our very different worldviews.

For instance, the monks seemed to see little utility in confidentiality. The abbot asked, puzzled, "How can the community help if we all don't know everything that is happening with one of our people?" A thought of my HIPAA training made me wince. "Everybody knows what everybody else is doing." That openness included health issues, mental health issues. Everything.

The abbot then suggested that we could perform health and mental health treatment in the temple. He could identify people with physical disease or mental disorders, and I could treat them right there: clinic in temple. The problem of boundaries and overlapping functions was entirely unfamiliar to him—and unclear even after we discussed it.

In fact, his whole concept of disease was quite different from mine. For him, disease is more of a spiritual state than a physiological one. *Samsara* is the continuous flow of birth, life, and death, filled with *dukkha*, or suffering. The cure to suffering is following the "Middle Path," or a spiritually balanced life. Health comes from following "…the Middle Path, which makes one both see and know, which leads to peace, to discernment, to enlightenment, to Nirvana" [1]. They don't teach that in American medical schools.

"Don't worry, Doctor." He smiled. "We can convince the peoples. Then you can make them *sok sabay*." Happy healthy.

I remember thinking how challenging it would be to reconcile such different cultures as we walked out of the temple back into the open air. The Western ideal of individualism, so praised in my medical ethics that it is protected in laws and codes celebrating autonomy and privacy, clashed against an Eastern ideal of collectivism, so celebrated by the Khmer people that it shaped human experience.

My senses still reeled from a flood of Khmer ethnic images, as though I had been transported to Angkor Wat for an hour. I felt as though the cultures could not clash more obviously.

And then I saw Jesus.

Jesus Christ was walking down the sidewalk, a cross on his back and a crown of thorns on his head. Roman soldiers were on all sides of him with whips and chains. A congregation of wailing mourners followed. For a moment, it seemed clear that I was amid a bizarre dream with amazing religious overtones.

And then it dawned on me that it was the Catholic holiday of *Viernes Santo*, Good Friday, and we were in a neighborhood heavily influenced by Mexican immigrants. "Jesus and the Romans" were performing *La Via Crucis*, the Way of the Cross, a procession in which an actor portraying Christ bears a cross down a street.

More bewildered than I, the monks looked at the scene with shock. *Why is a bloody man in shackles carrying an enormous piece of wood along our sidewalk and getting whipped by Mexican gladiators?*

And the Christian congregation looked back at the monks with wonder. *Why are these orange-robed Asians with shaved heads and eyebrows standing in the way of our sacred procession?*

The Way of the Cross passed right through the Middle Path, if you will.

As the Christians moved past, the Buddhist abbot asked, "Who is that?"

"That?" I responded, not really sure how to start. "Oh, that. Well, that's Jesus Christ."

The monk paused. And he then leaned in close, as if trying to get in on a secret. "Who is...Jesus Christ?"

He had never heard of Him.

San Jose, USA   Daryn Reicherter
Good Friday and Magha Puja, 2007

Reference

1. Kornfield, J., editor. The teachings of the Buddha. Adapted from the Samyutta Nikaya. Boston: Shambala Publications; 1993, p. 30.

Acknowledgments

The editors wish to thank the many contributing authors who generously shared hypothetical cases and real-life dilemmas for inclusion in the *Professionalism and Ethics in Medicine: A Study Guide for Physicians and Physicians-in-Training*. The authors, listed alphabetically, are Richard Balon, M.D.; Victor G. Carrion, M.D.; Jodi K. Casados, M.D.; John H. Coverdale, M.D., M.Ed.; Kristi R. Estabrook, M.D.; Cynthia M. A. Geppert, M.D.; M.P.H., Ph.D.; Michelle Goldsmith, M.D., M.A.; Shaili Jain, M.D.; Joseph B. Layde, M.D., J.D.; Sermsak Lolak, M.D.; Celeste Lopez, M.D.; Steven B. McCann, M.D.; Teresita A. McCarty, M.D.; Lawrence B. McCullough, Ph.D.; Lawrence M. McGlynn, M.D.; Christine Moutier, M.D.; Joshua Reiher, M.D.; Richard Shaw, M.D.; Christopher Warner, M.D., LTC; and Mark T. Wright, M.D. We also thank our chapter authors, Elias Aboujaoude, M.D., M.A.; John H. Coverdale, M.D., M.Ed.; Shashank V. Joshi, M.D.; Jane Paik Kim, Ph.D.; Joseph B. Layde, M.D., J.D.; Lawrence B. McCullough, Ph.D.; Maurice M. Ohayon, M.D., D.Sc., Ph.D.; and Andres J. Pumariega, M.D.

We especially express our appreciation to Josh Reiher, M.D., who helped in careful revisions of the case-based questions and narratives while a medical student and resident physician.

The editors and authors sincerely thank Ann Tennier, ELS, editorial associate extraordinaire, who brings a generous intellect and a generous heart to every collaboration. We also thank Megan Cid; Melinda Hantke; Thomas W. Heinrich, M.D.; Madeline McDonald Lane-McKinley, Ph.D. (cand.); and Kevin Wright for their assistance at various stages in the preparation of the book.

The editors and authors also wish to thank Richard Lansing of Springer Science+Business Media, LLC, a gentleman who has shown himself at every turn to be a wonderful colleague and publisher.

Contents

Contributors

Elias Aboujaoude, M.D., M.A. Department of Psychiatry and Behavioral Sciences, Stanford University School of Medicine, Stanford, CA, USA

Richard Balon, M.D. Department of Psychiatry and Behavioral Neurosciences, Wayne State University School of Medicine, Detroit, MI, USA

Victor G. Carrion, M.D. Department of Psychiatry and Behavioral Sciences, Stanford University School of Medicine, Stanford, CA, USA

Jodi K. Casados, M.D. Presbyterian Medical Group, Espanola, NM, USA

John H. Coverdale, M.D., M.Ed. Menninger Department of Psychiatry and Behavioral Sciences, Baylor College of Medicine, Houston, TX, USA

Kristi Estabrook, M.D. Department of Psychiatry and Behavioral Medicine, Medical College of Wisconsin, Milwaukee, WI, USA

Cynthia M.A. Geppert, M.D., M.P.H., Ph.D., Department of Psychiatry, University of New Mexico School of Medicine, New Mexico Veterans Affairs Health Care System, Albuquerque, NM, USA

Michelle Goldsmith, M.D., M.A. Department of Psychiatry and Behavioral Sciences, Division of Child and Adolescent Psychiatry, Stanford University School of Medicine, Stanford, CA, USA

Shaili Jain, M.D. Department of Psychiatry and Behavioral Sciences, Stanford University School of Medicine, Stanford, CA, USA

Shashank V. Joshi, M.D. Department of Psychiatry and Behavioral Sciences, Stanford University School of Medicine, Stanford, CA, USA

Jane Paik Kim, Ph.D. Department of Psychiatry and Behavorial Sciences, Stanford University School of Medicine, Stanford, CA, USA

Joseph B. Layde, M.D., J.D. Department of Psychiatry and Behavioral Medicine, Medical College of Wisconsin, Milwaukee, WI, USA

Sermsak Lolak, M.D. Department of Psychiatry and Behavioral Sciences, The George Washington University School of Medicine and Health Sciences, Washington, DC, USA

Celeste Lopez, M.D. Department of Psychiatry and Behavioral Sciences, Stanford University School of Medicine, Stanford, CA, USA

Steven B. McCann, M.D. Department of Obstetrics and Gynecology, Elmbrook Memorial Hospital, Brookfield, WI, USA

Teresita A. McCarty, M.D. Department of Psychiatry, University of New Mexico School of Medicine, Albuquerque, NM, USA

Lawrence B. McCullough, Ph.D. Center for Medical Ethics and Health Policy, Baylor College of Medicine, Houston, TX, USA

Lawrence M. McGlynn, M.D. Department of Psychiatry and Behavioral Sciences, Stanford University, Stanford, CA, USA

Christine Moutier, M.D. American Foundation for Suicide Prevention, New York, NY, USA

Maurice M. Ohayon, M.D., D.Sc., Ph.D. Department of Psychiatry and Behavorial Science, Division of Public Mental Health and Population Sciences, Stanford University School of Medicine, Stanford, CA, USA

Andres J. Pumariega, M.D. Department of Psychiatry, Cooper Health System and Cooper Medical School Of Rowan University, Camden, NJ, USA

Daryn Reicherter, M.D. Department of Psychiatry and Behavorial Sciences, Stanford University School of Medicine, Stanford, CA, USA

Joshua Reiher, M.D. Saint Anthony North Hospital, Westminster, CO, USA

Laura Weiss Roberts, M.D., M.A. Department of Psychiatry and Behavioral Sciences, Stanford University School of Medicine, Stanford, CA, USA

Richard J. Shaw, M.D. Department of Psychiatry and Behavorial Sciences, Stanford University School of Medicine, Stanford, CA, USA

Christopher H. Warner, M.D., LTC Department of Behavioral Medicine, Blanchfield Army Community Hospital, Fort Campbell State, KY, USA

Mark T. Wright, M.D. Departments of Psychiatry and Behavioral Medicine and Neurology, Medical College of Wisconsin, Milwaukee, WI, USA

Part I
Foundations

Chapter 1
Introduction to Ethics in Clinical Medicine

Elias Aboujaoude, Laura Weiss Roberts, and Daryn Reicherter

It is common to think of ethics in medicine as an ossified set of dictates – or, alternatively, as an innate, intuitive skill that one either possesses or does not. Yet a look at how the field has evolved, the lessons learned, and the changing nature of the challenges faced make clear that biomedical ethics is a dynamic, applied, scholarly discipline. Moreover, biomedical ethics is a discipline rooted in enduring principles that relate to the fundamental human experiences of suffering and healing and may be learned and taught.

Physicians are professionals entrusted by society to develop and use their expertise to serve others – to improve the health of individual patients, families, and entire communities. In this life of service, physicians as clinicians, biomedical scientists, and teachers and their earlier-career colleagues in training are called upon to fulfill the ethical standards of the medical and scientific professions. When viewed in the abstract, this requirement may appear straightforward and perhaps easy – the combination of traditions, rules, and common sense *should* suffice. History humbles us, however. Imagine the complexity faced by the medical field just a few decades ago as it extended the boundaries of life in the care of extremely low-birth-weight infants, established a new definition for brain death, developed innovative transplantation methods, grappled with fair allocation of scarce organs, and struggled through the question of the moral equivalency of withdrawing and withholding life support as new technology was introduced to intensive medical care.

E. Aboujaoude, M.D., M.A. • L.W. Roberts, M.D., M.A. (✉) • D. Reicherter, M.D.
Department of Psychiatry and Behavioral Sciences, Stanford University
School of Medicine, Stanford, CA, USA
e-mail: RobertsL@stanford.edu

© Springer Science+Business Media New York 2015
L.W. Roberts, D. Reicherter (eds.), *Professionalism and Ethics in Medicine*,
DOI 10.1007/978-1-4939-1686-3_1

In the current era of Institutional Review Boards, the Tuskegee Syphilis Study, conducted between 1932 and 1972 to study the progression of untreated syphilis in rural black men in Alabama, is now rightly viewed as a horrifying example of abuse of the researcher-subject power differential [1]. Thanks to increased awareness of, and appreciation for, the importance of medical ethics, it is nearly incomprehensible today how the US Public Health Service, which oversaw the study, could have allowed the experiment to proceed for nearly 25 years after penicillin became a widely used and effective treatment for syphilis. The Human Radiation Experiments, also conducted by the US government over decades and in a manner that placed disproportionate burden on distinct ethnic/racial minority groups in southwestern United States, serve as another grave example of enduring and broadly based exploitative research [2]. One explanation for these tragedies is that very bad people did these very terrible things, and there may be substantial truth to this. Yet the widespread conduct of what we now view as appallingly unethical clinical research, as documented in the landmark *New England Journal of Medicine* report by Henry K. Beecher in 1966 [3], reveals that well-intentioned professionals will do things that are later understood to be wrong. Similarly, our behavior today will be viewed in the harsh light of tomorrow. For this reason, the need to educate physicians and scientists about the ethical lessons of the past and to prepare them for emerging challenges is absolute. It is our hope and expectation that trainees and researchers who are formally taught about ethics and instructed in applying ethical skills, as can happen through Accreditation Council for Graduate Medical Education core competency and other classes, are more likely to be attuned to new ethical tensions as they arise and more likely to prevent another Tuskegee.

There is no shortage of new challenges and potential pitfalls, making formal biomedical ethics training a necessity for physicians and physicians-in-training. For example, given diminishing resources and rising costs, how do we in society balance the use of expensive medications and life support tools that can extend the life of patients with irreversible brain damage alongside the need to treat millions of uninsured patients who cannot afford even basic medical care? How do we guarantee patient confidentiality as we race to adopt electronic health records and consider national health identifiers? How do we avoid the eugenics trap as we use genetic testing to diagnose predisposition to illness and genetic manipulation to prevent disease? As more innovative procedures get tested in a broadening range of disorders, how do we guarantee a fair informed consent process when conducting experiments with potentially vulnerable research volunteers?

Approaching biomedical ethics as a "living" discipline—one that draws from a rich tradition and learns from past failings as it informs present-day actions and stances—can help answer such questions while protecting patient/subject and practitioner/investigator and while helping ensure a morally competent profession that lives up to the great trust and privileges bestowed upon it. Such an approach assumes familiarity with, and application of, some core principles of biomedical ethics and some essential ethical skills. Rather than innate or purely intuitive, these principles and skills can be studied, internalized, and continuously applied and refined throughout one's career.

Biomedical ethics is not only a "living" discipline; it is also a discipline with a developmental history and evolutionary arc. It has been alive for centuries. Today's ethical questions are usually not unlike ancient moral questions, with a rich tradition of thought, discourse, and debate echoing through history. The basis of contemporary ethics resides in philosophy, religion, and law. These traditions must be acknowledged to appreciate the complexity of contemporary reasoning in biomedical ethics.

Biomedical ethics is a subset of the philosophy of ethics, a tradition that spans most of written history and draws from human experience as well as social sciences and philosophy, religion, and law. This intrinsically interdisciplinary field has evolved with important historical innovations and breakthroughs. Medical traditions from distinct parts of the world have evolved largely independently. In this chapter, we focus on the evolution and tradition in the Western civilization only. Physicians can benefit from familiarizing themselves with legal issues, the evolution of the non-Western traditions of medical ethics, and issues pertaining to cultural humility and sensitivity as explored in the chapters that follow.

By the fourth-century BC, medical ethics and professionalism were active topics in the work of physicians and the writings of philosophers. The Hippocratic Oath (Box 1.1), which focuses on professionalism and ethical responsibility, has become a cherished doctrine among many Western physicians and is commonly recited in the graduation ceremonies of medical schools in the United States. The Oath's themes, simple and relevant, permeate many chapters in this and other books about Western medical ethics.

Formal codes for ethics in medicine over hundreds of years since the time of Hippocrates have continued to redefine and refine physician ethics and professional standards. The first major written formal code of medical ethics is *Formula Comitis Archiatrorum*, written in the fifth century and preserved in the work of Cassiodorus [4]. This document highlights the need for deepening knowledge and consultation, which remain contemporary themes of professionalism. The philosophy of Thomas Percival (late eighteenth century) is also foundational to modern medical ethical codes. In his work *Medical Ethics or a Code of Institutes and Percepts, Adapted to Professional Conduct of Physicians and Surgeons* [5], he set ethical standards for physicians that are foundational for medical practitioners today. His work was highly influential for creating modern standards for medical ethical thinking, public health, and the right to medical care. During the same era that Percival developed codes of conduct for physicians, trends toward adopting official standards began to become more common. In 1815, the Apothecaries Act was established in England to regulate standards for physicians.

Beyond these formal codes establishing ethical standards, themes from religious texts and the work of moral philosophers have shaped thinking about the profession of medicine and the moral duties of physicians. For example, in his *Practical Ethics of the Physician* [6], Ali al-Ruhawi, a ninth-century Arab physician and philosopher, argued that physicians should be subject to peer review, a notion that has endured. The influence of great moral philosophers and theologians, including Maimonides, Immanuel Kant, and Thomas Aquinas, is felt throughout modern biomedical ethics.

Box 1.1 Hippocratic Oath [7]

I swear to fulfill, to the best of my ability and judgment, this covenant:

I will respect the hard-won scientific gains of those physicians in whose steps I walk, and gladly share such knowledge as is mine with those who are to follow.

I will apply, for the benefit of the sick, all measures [that] are required, avoiding those twin traps of overtreatment and therapeutic nihilism.

I will remember that there is art to medicine as well as science, and that warmth, sympathy, and understanding may outweigh the surgeon's knife or the chemist's drug.

I will not be ashamed to say "I know not," nor will I fail to call in my colleagues when the skills of another are needed for a patient's recovery.

I will respect the privacy of my patients, for their problems are not disclosed to me that the world may know. Most especially must I tread with care in matters of life and death. If it is given me to save a life, all thanks. But it may also be within my power to take a life; this awesome responsibility must be faced with great humbleness and awareness of my own frailty. Above all, I must not play at God.

I will remember that I do not treat a fever chart, a cancerous growth, but a sick human being, whose illness may affect the person's family and economic stability. My responsibility includes these related problems, if I am to care adequately for the sick.

I will prevent disease whenever I can, for prevention is preferable to cure.

I will remember that I remain a member of society, with special obligations to all my fellow human beings, those sound of mind and body as well as the infirm.

If I do not violate this oath, may I enjoy life and art, respected while I live and remembered with affection thereafter. May I always act so as to preserve the finest traditions of my calling and may I long experience the joy of healing those who seek my help.

Modern Ethical Codes for Physicians

The American Medical Association (AMA) adopted a first code of ethical conduct for physicians in 1847. The AMA Principles of Medical Ethics [8] has served as an authoritative guide on honorable behavior for doctors, and its four revisions reflect the evolution of clinical medicine over time [9]. The preamble to the 2001 revision points to a unique role for the physician in society, one with broad responsibilities that come with the privilege of belonging to the profession: The "physician must recognize responsibility to patients first and foremost, as well as to society, to other health professionals, and to self" [8]. Like previous versions, the 2001 preamble also emphasizes that the "Principles adopted by the American Medical Association are not laws, but standards of conduct" [8], thereby highlighting the positive imperative to act not just within the sometimes narrower legal definition but also morally.

Medical subspecialties and other health-related groups have felt the same need to codify what constitutes ethical behavior for their members. The American Board of Internal Medicine has helped develop a very thoughtful "Physician Charter" related to the ethical and professional duties of physicians [10], as has the American Board of Pediatrics [11]. The American College of Physicians [12] has published position papers on several "hot button" ethical topics to help its members and the general public navigate the issues at play. Topics addressed in the individual position papers include end-of-life care, health right as a human right, the ethics of managed care, the ethics of using human subjects in research, and the ethics of physician-industry relations. Others organizations that have emphasized moral behavior for their members and have published guidelines to promote and define it include the American Psychiatric Association [13], the American College of Surgeons [14], the American Heart Association [15], the College of American Pathologists [16], the American Academy of Dermatology [17], the American Psychological Association [18], the American Pharmacists Association [19], the American Nurses Association [20], and the National Association of Social Workers [21].

Ethical Codes for Biomedical Researchers

"The voluntary consent of the human subject is absolutely essential," thus begins the Nuremberg Code [22], the famous document on medical research ethics developed after World War II in response to Nazi experimentation with humans. Other components of the Code include the need to refrain from conducting research if there is reason to believe it might lead to death or disability, avoidance of unnecessary suffering to participants, need to weigh the degree of risk against the importance of the research question, and usefulness to society of the research's results and their unattainability by other means. The two other foundational documents in the history of medical research ethics are the World Medical Association's Declaration of Helsinki [23] and the Belmont Report [24], published by the National Commission for the Protection of Human Subjects of Biomedical and Behavioral Research. The Declaration of Helsinki expanded on the Nuremberg Code, highlighting privacy safeguards, environmental protections, the ethics of placebo use, and the moral duties of authors and publishers, including the duty to publish negative findings and declare sources of funding and potential conflicts of interest. The Belmont Report distinguished between "practice" (meant solely to enhance well-being by using interventions with reasonable success rates) and "research" (meant to test a hypothesis and contribute to general knowledge), and it elaborated on *respect for persons, beneficence*, and *justice* as three principles essential to ethical research.

Early-career physicians naturally will wonder how it is ever ethical to "use" a human being as the "subject" of research, just as they may struggle with this same question in "using" patients to learn their profession. There are some opinion leaders who hold that these endeavors will never be ethical and that they are, by definition, exploitative. There are other opinion leaders, however, who believe that it may be possible to invite well-informed and authentic voluntary participation in human studies. The participation of these individuals in research is grounded in honesty and mutualism. The scientist's responsibility in this situation is to be rigorous, to invite volunteers for whom the question at hand is relevant, to safeguard against unnecessary risks, to behave with integrity, and to advance the field through what is learned.

In perhaps another example of evolving ethical sensibilities, the use of animals in research has become the topic of increased attention. Animal research ethics principles give emphasis to minimizing the use of animals and minimizing the distress and discomfort of animals in research. The "three Rs" of animal research ethics are reduction (of the number of animals used), refinement (of procedures to minimize pain, suffering, distress), and replacement (e.g., by nonanimal models) [25], and all animal research must be performed in order to answer a question of importance to society to be ethically acceptable. Although animal research is seen as an ethical dilemma, the majority of those who respond to public opinion surveys (greater than 80 % according to various surveys) support animal research if it meets the following criteria: it targets serious medical purposes, animal suffering is minimized, and alternatives to animal use are explored [26]. The surveys also suggest a desire by the public to limit cosmetic testing in animals and to implement a supervisory "quality control" mechanism that helps ensure animal welfare. Attempts have been made to delineate standards for research in animals. The American Psychological Association's Committee on Animal Research and Care, for example, published guidelines for use by its members who conduct such research, requiring them to "comply with APA ethical standards in the treatment of their sample, human or animal" [27].

Core Bioethical Principles

A handful of crucial bioethics principles have traditionally defined the moral basis of clinical care and research. These principles are *autonomy*, *beneficence*, *nonmaleficence*, *respect for persons*, *confidentiality*, *justice*, and *veracity*. If each patient or study volunteer situation represented, from an ethical point of view, a simple exercise in doing good (*beneficence*) or telling the truth (*veracity*) or honoring preferences (*autonomy*), there would be little controversy and little to discuss. Ethical tensions do not arise when the "right thing to do" is obvious, as occurs when a positive and a negative are apparent and are pitted against each other. Rather, dilemmas emerge, usually, when two "good things" are in conflict (Table 1.1).

Table 1.1 Ethical tensions in common clinical situations

Clinical situation	Relevant ethical principles	Conflicts and tensions
A patient refuses a medically indicated treatment	*Autonomy* and *beneficence*	The patient's right to make his or her own decisions is in tension with the physician's duty to do good by providing medically indicated treatment
A patient tells his psychiatrist that he plans to harm another person	*Confidentiality* and *beneficence*	The physician's duty to guard his patient's privacy must be balanced against the obligation to protect the threatened third party
A close friend asks a psychiatrist to write a prescription for a sleep medicine	*Nonmaleficence*	The desire to oblige a friend may conflict with the psychiatrist's duty to avoid harm by prescribing without conducting a thorough medical evaluation and establishing a treatment relationship
The parent of an adolescent patient asks the psychiatrist for information about the patient's sexual activity and drug or alcohol use	*Confidentiality* and *beneficence*	The psychiatrist's duty to guard his patient's privacy may be in tension with the psychiatrist's desire to do good by educating the parent about the child's high-risk behaviors
A patient asks a psychiatrist to document a less stigmatizing diagnosis when filling out insurance forms	*Veracity* and *nonmaleficence*	The psychiatrist's obligation to document the truth may be in tension with the desire to avoid the harm that may occur if the insurance company learns of the diagnosis
A psychiatrist is sexually attracted to a patient	*Fidelity* and *nonmaleficence*	Sexual activity with a patient violates the psychiatrist's obligation to remain faithful to the goals of treatment and the duty to avoid harming the patient by sexual exploitation
A rural patient needs a treatment the psychiatrist is not competent to provide; no other practitioner is available	*Nonmaleficence*	The psychiatrist's duty to avoid harming the patient by practicing outside his scope of competencies is in conflict with the obligation to avoid harming the patient by leaving him without any treatment provider
A medical student performs a lumbar puncture for the first time on a patient	*Nonmaleficence* and *beneficence*	The medical student's obligation to avoid harming the patient by performing a procedure without sufficient expertise must be balanced against the student's need to learn by doing in order to help future patients

(continued)

Table 1.1 (continued)

Clinical situation	Relevant ethical principles	Conflicts and tensions
A psychiatrist treating a physician believes the patient is too impaired to practice medicine safely; the patient/physician refuses to close his practice because he has no other source of income	*Confidentiality, nonmaleficence,* and *beneficence*	The psychiatrist's duty to guard his patient's privacy and to avoid harming him is in tension with the obligation to protect the impaired physician's patients by reporting the impairment to the proper authorities
A pharmaceutical company offers a psychiatrist an unusually large fee for referring patients to a research trial	*Fidelity*	Financial self-interest threatens the psychiatrist's duty to remain faithful to the goals of treatment and to the role of healer
A psychiatrist transfers the care of a difficult patient to another provider	*Fidelity, nonmaleficence,* and *beneficence*	The psychiatrist's obligations to remain faithful to the goals of treatment and to avoid the harm of patient abandonment must be balanced against the duty to do good by transferring care to a more competent or appropriate provider when clinically necessary

Reprinted with permission from Concise Guide to Ethics in Mental Health Care, (Copyright ©2004) and Professionalism and Ethics: Q & A Self-Study Guide for Mental Health Professionals (Copyright ©2008). American Psychiatric Association

Stated differently, instead of presenting themselves one at a time, two or more of these principles may simultaneously be at play, creating the possibility of tension and failure, with negative consequences to those involved.

Autonomy

Informed Consent, Advance Directives, Alternative Decision-Making

The reasons for which patients may refuse their doctors' recommended treatments are varied and include cultural or religious prohibitions (e.g., against accepting blood transfusions); an exaggerated sense of understanding of their illness and what works best for it (sometimes colored by variable-quality information gleaned online or through direct-to-consumer marketing); or the illness itself (as can happen in patients with disorders affecting the brain). Consider the patient with pancreatic cancer who initially presents with painless jaundice and weight loss and with neuropsychiatric sequelae of the disease – dysphoria, despair, amotivation, and nihilism about the future. Any expressed preference by the patient to refuse recommended treatment should be viewed as *both* a possible authentic statement of the patient's personal wishes *and* a possible clinical sign of underlying disease that warrants treatment. Several ethical duties of the physician emerge in this situation. The physician must seek to do good, avoid harm, honor the patient's wishes, and demonstrate regard for the patient's humanity and dignity. If each of these duties "compete" equally, then it is difficult to find resolution. Placing primacy on clarifying the exact nature of the clinical situation and establishing a therapeutic alliance in which the goals for treatment can be defined in a time-sensitive (but not an immediate, "all or nothing") manner will often allow for a greater harmony of these ethical duties.

Consider a second example that illustrates the nuances in informed consent, and informed refusal, in ethical patient care. A woman has a debilitating case of panic disorder that renders her incapable of working or maintaining meaningful social relationships [28]. In addition to many excessive worries, it is not uncommon for such a patient also to fear that medications might make her worse and to prefer the level of misery she is in over the possibility of side effects that might exacerbate her condition. This fear might drive her to reject a recommended medication trial that has a good chance of alleviating her anxiety. The doctor-patient dynamic in such a case illustrates the ethical concept of *autonomy*, defined as "self-rule" or the ability to make reasoned decisions for oneself and act on the basis of such decisions. Informed consent serves as the cornerstone of ethical practice in clinical and research settings. In this example, the physician's duty to recommend psychopharmacological treatment to someone who is unlikely to improve otherwise is in tension with the obligation to respect patient *autonomy*. If the physician determines that the patient has decisional capacity to refuse the recommended treatment, the most ethically sound response would be to honor the patient's preference and to define with the patient the circumstances under which the physician would like to revisit the decision in the future.

The assessment regarding decisional capacity rests on whether four standards are met [29–32]: (a) the ability to communicate unambiguously one's preference; (b) an understanding of the information needed to reach the specific decision (in this case an understanding of the potential for positive and negative outcomes with the recommended intervention); (c) an appreciation of symptom severity and the resulting impairment, insight about the disease process, as well as an appreciation of the nature of this decision in the context of one's life; and (d) the ability to reason, by which is meant the capacity to weigh information, consider alternatives, and understand the consequence of no treatment at all. In the court system, the abilities to understand and to reason are valued most highly in informed consent (and refusal) cases, although, in clinical practice, these abilities are often viewed as necessary but not sufficient and the appreciation and insight with which the patient approaches the situation have greater importance. Within the field of biomedical research, a sound informed consent process takes on meaning beyond the protection of human volunteers. It is crucial for earning and maintaining public trust in research – now under increased strain and scrutiny [33, 34].

The same deference to the bioethical principle of patient *autonomy* is the basis of policies regarding advance directives and alternative decision-making. In cases when an individual is found, via a clinical or legal determination, to lack decisional capacity, an advance directive, in the form of a document that specifies an individual's wishes about future care or the presence of a surrogate or alternative decision-maker previously appointed by the individual, can be invaluable in directing care. There are two medicolegal standards for alternative decision-makers: what is referred to as the "substituted judgment" standard, in which the surrogate decision-maker endeavors to make the decision that most closely aligns with an understanding of what the patient would want, and what is referred to as the "best interests" standard, in which the surrogate decision-maker based on what he believes is in the best interests of the patient. Most states have implemented the "substituted judgment" standard in an effort to honor the *autonomy* of the patient. Wise and thoughtful practitioners in clinical medicine also work to incorporate the preferences of the patient, to the extent it is possible, in the treatment plan. In other words, the patient may not be capable of the "big decisions" in his or her care but should be included in whatever "smaller decisions" are possible.

The growing adoption of advance directives and alternative decision-making and the growing emphasis that a discussion about them takes place between patient and practitioner reflect increased appreciation for *autonomy* as a cornerstone of medical care, one that remains highly relevant even if physical or mental illness compromises the patient.

Beneficence Versus Nonmaleficence, Veracity, Justice

A medical student performing his first lumbar puncture or a surgery resident performing her first hernia repair is an example that highlights the tension in *beneficence* and *nonmaleficence* in clinical training settings [35]. On one hand, there is potential for harm resulting to the patient due to the student's or resident's inexperience. On the other hand, there is undeniable good to be gained from a new generation of doctors able to perform essential medical procedures on future patients. The student's or trainee's obligation to avoid harming a patient by performing an invasive procedure without adequate practice has to be balanced against the need to "learn by doing" as this is the only way to "become" an experienced doctor and gain the necessary expertise. The principle of *nonmaleficence*, defined as the duty to avoid doing harm, is in conflict here with the principle of *beneficence*, or the obligation to benefit patients and seek their good.

An adequate resolution to this typical medical school and residency-training situation is for the student or trainee to study and demonstrate an "abstract" understanding of the procedure in question, to observe an adequate number of similar procedures being performed by experienced practitioners, and then to obtain informed consent from the patient to perform the procedure under close and competent supervision. Truthfulness with the patient who often is aware of the hospital as a teaching setting – a component of *veracity*, discussed in more detail below – is critical to the foundation of the therapeutic relationship in this situation and to the public trust more broadly. From our experience, we believe that the physician-in-training will encounter another important ethical principle that is witnessed all of the time in clinical settings: *altruism*. The deep generosity of patients who authentically provide consent for treatment in training settings can be stunning. With every action taken and decision made, everyday medical practice brings healthcare professionals countless opportunities to maximize the good and minimize the harm and to be truthful and honorable in engaging patients who live out the consequences of these decisions.

Upholding the principle of *beneficence* in a way that causes the most good to be done for the most people can also help ensure that the ethical principle of *justice* is respected. *Justice* in bioethics represents fairness and equitability in the distribution of resources and burdens throughout society. It is increasingly factoring into health-care policy in a manner that reflects evolving societal appreciation for its impor-tance. As an example, the need for *justice* in medical coverage is translating into legislation that is gradually outlawing the two-tier insurance model whereby mental health and substance addiction problems could be treated less generously than other disorders. For instance, the Mental Health Parity and Addiction Equity Act, which took effect in 2010 [36], requires that group health plans that include mental health and substance use disorder benefits along with standard medical coverage must treat them equally in terms of out-of-pocket costs, benefit limits, prior authorization requirements, and utilization review standards. According to this Act, the insurer should demand the same level of scientific evidence for mental health and substance use treatment as for medical and surgical benefits.

Keeping in mind the idea of distributive *justice*, the positive value of *veracity*, and the principles of *beneficence* and *nonmaleficence* while weighing actions and decisions can help ensure that healthcare professionals remain a positive force in their patients' lives and in society at large.

Respect for Persons

Caring for the "Difficult Patient"

Whether clear to them or unconscious, medical professionals carry preferences and prejudices, and those can influence the care they provide, sometimes negatively, as in the case of the "difficult patient" [37]. When substance abuse, criminal history, a personality disorder, opposing political views, or homelessness complicates a physical or psychological problem, the result can be an exasperating patient who is a "setup" for ethical violations. Consider the patient who implies to her 70-something-year-old cardiologist that he is not up to date on cardiology advances and, thus, that she doubts he can help her or inform her of new treatment options; or the patient who signals to his female surgeon that a male surgeon would be more dexterous with his hands; or the patient who voices to her nurse racist views about previous nurses assigned to her, expressing relief at "finally" working with someone who looked like her. Ageism, sexism, racism, and other problematic views or behaviors held or displayed by patients do not constitute a carte blanche to terminate treatment, refer out, or provide suboptimal care. If the patient in these examples decides to continue to seek care from the older doctor, the female doctor, or the racially diverse hospital – and many will for lack of alternatives acceptable to them – it is the doctor's and nurse's duty to continue to be the best providers they can be. For despite the considerable negative reaction and exhaustion such patients often engender, the obligation to deliver competent care is not suspended, and the patient still enjoys innate worth and deserves genuine consideration.

These observations derive from the core bioethical principle of *respect for persons*, which represents the virtue of according intrinsic value to the individual. Giving inadequate treatment to an established patient, subtly encouraging the patient to seek care elsewhere, and terminating treatment altogether all constitute patient abandonment from an ethical perspective and represent a failure to fulfill the duty to demonstrate *respect for persons*. These actions may also directly or indirectly harm the patient's well-being. *Respect for persons* requires that the well-being of the patient be served without judgment and preconception and with regard for the patient's dignity, despite provocation or personal antipathy.

Heightened self-awareness and self-care on the part of the clinician, as well as appropriate consultation, can help prevent provider exhaustion and ethical compromises while working with the "difficult patient." To help achieve that goal, one of us (LWR) has suggested a three-step approach [38]. First, recognize what makes a patient problematic (e.g., "med-seeking behavior," noncompliance with recommendations, "manipulative" style). Second, view the "difficult" behavior as a clinical sign or as symptom with a differential diagnosis (e.g., the patient's irritability may be a manifestation of substance withdrawal). Third, pause before reacting to "triggers." This is easier if we in medicine remind ourselves that the difficult patient is, above all, a patient who is suffering. By continuing to help allay this patient's pain, physicians are upholding the bioethical principle of *respect for persons*.

Confidentiality and Veracity

Nondisclosure Versus Honest Disclosure

Confidentiality has formed a centerpiece of medical practice and the doctor-patient relationship over centuries. Defined as the obligation not to disclose information obtained from patients or observed about them without their permission, *confidentiality* has been an established duty of physicians at least since Hippocrates wrote: "What I may see or hear in the course of treatment … in regard to the life of men … I will keep to myself, holding such things to be shameful to be spoken about" [39].

Only extraordinary circumstances – usually as defined by local law – suspend this duty. Examples include suspected child or elder abuse and imminent threat to a third party. In the latter case, *confidentiality* is trumped by the duty to protect members of the public from a patient's violent intentions, as demonstrated in *Tarasoff v Regents of the University of California, 1974 and 1976* [40].

New applications of the notion of *confidentiality* are, in part, at the origin of the 1996 Health Insurance Portability and Accountability Act [41] and the modern dictate that electronic health information be protected behind secure passwords that are changed frequently. Yet as health professionals strive to uphold *confidentiality* in the age of cyber leaks and identity theft, it is imperative to educate patients about the safeguards – new and old – that are in place for the protection of their private information, because fear about losing control over health records continues to cause patients to avoid or delay seeking treatment.

If *confidentiality* entails nondisclosure, the principle of *veracity* reflects a duty to be honest and not engage in deception when disclosure does occur. As it relates to patients, *veracity* surpasses simply not lying to them to include a positive duty to provide the whole truth, not only the selective pieces that the patient may prefer to hear. When it comes to sharing health information with other "approved" entities, such as medical or life insurance companies, *veracity* implies an obligation to tell the truth even if it contradicts the patient's wishes, as in the example of the patient who asks the doctor to document a less stigmatizing diagnosis or one that is more likely to be granted insurance coverage. This said, the physician must use judgment – providing only the information necessary and required to fulfill the obligation. When patients are the victims of sexual assault, for example, *confidentiality* may be delimited by local law enforcement, who require information in order to pursue the attacker. In this situation, medical personnel in the emergency department should not turn over the patient's chart or electronic records for indiscriminant perusal – breaches of *confidentiality*, in fact, most typically occur as inadvertent disclosures in the context of appropriate disclosures with narrower scope. Carefully managing the flow of private information at the disposition of medical professionals – knowing when to withhold and when to truthfully share – is a core ethical duty that is only becoming more relevant as the Information Age reinvents how health professionals generate, consume, store, and relay information.

Essential Ethical Skills

Six skills are essential for ethical problem solving in the health professional (Table 1.2). These skills are especially salient in psychiatry because of the increased vulnerability of mentally ill patients and the fact that psychiatric illness often alters insight and thinking patterns. For these reasons, moral dilemmas are often magnified in mental healthcare and research. But no medical discipline is immune to

Table 1.2 Essential ethics skills in clinical practice

The ability to identify the ethical features of a patient's care
The ability to see how one's own life experiences, attitudes, and knowledge may influence one's care of a patient
The ability to identify one's areas of clinical expertise (i.e., scope of clinical competence) and to work within those boundaries
The ability to anticipate ethically risky or problematic situations
The ability to gather additional information and to seek consultation and additional expertise in order to clarify and, ideally, resolve the conflict
The ability to build additional ethical safeguards into the patient care situation

Reprinted with permission from Concise Guide to Ethics in Mental Health Care, (Copyright ©2004) and Professionalism and Ethics: Q & A Self-Study Guide for Mental Health Professionals (Copyright ©2008). American Psychiatric Association

difficult ethical dilemmas, and any medical provider or researcher could benefit from acquiring and nurturing the six skills they highlight: [1] recognizing ethical issues as they arise, [2] understanding how personal values affect the care one delivers, [3] seeing the limits of one's knowledge, [4] seeking consultation around ethical issues, [5] identifying high-risk situations more likely to produce ethical conflicts, and [6] incorporating ethical safeguards into one's work.

The first essential ethical skill is the ability to recognize ethical issues as they arise. This recognition derives from intuition (the internal sense that "something isn't right"), education (familiarizing oneself with bioethical principles and systematically applying them), experience, or a combination. By educating themselves about these scenarios and learning to anticipate them, healthcare professionals can feel more confident about "doing the right thing" when faced with an ethical dilemma, thus supplementing their intuitive sense about what constitutes appropriate behavior in the ethically challenging situation.

The ability to understand how personal values, likes, and dislikes may influence care constitutes the second essential ethical skill. Sometimes these factors are obvious, such as the belligerent or aggressive patient who elicits fear and anger in an evaluating physician or a patient who has just "ruined" a transplanted organ by nonadherence to the posttransplant regimen or who has begun using substances (again). Sometimes these factors are not obvious, such as the patient who reminds one of one's Aunt Marge, child, or first boss or who come from a background very dissimilar to the physician's own. There is no blame in having complex reactions to patients – in fact, on one hand, these reactions can be great clinical tools and can serve a wise physician well as he or she comes to understand the "signal" received in the physician-patient interaction. On the other hand, remaining unaware and unthoughtful about these reactions can lead to prejudicial and downright poor treatment of patients who "fit" into these spots in one's personality. "Know thyself," applied to the practitioner, is a safeguard against preferential treatment for patients to whom we relate and inferior care for those of whom we disapprove. The concept of countertransference, first described in the psychiatric literature as "a result of the patient's influence on [the physician's] unconscious feelings" [42], is applicable across all fields of medicine. All medical professionals should take responsibility for a careful self-examination of how positive and, more important, negative feelings engendered by their patients can end up influencing the ethical integrity of their work.

A third ethical skill is awareness into the limits of one's expertise and a willingness to practice within those limits. Accepting and working within one's true capabilities can be challenging in situations such as in inner city and rural settings, where unreasonable demands are sometimes placed on the limited number of practitioners available. Practitioners there might be tempted to provide medical services for which they lack adequate training, not necessarily out of exaggerated self-confidence but for lack of other alternatives to the patient.

Consciousness into what falls within one's scope of practice, and the related fourth ethical skill of being willing to seek consultation around clinically and ethically difficult issues, can help mitigate some of the challenges. New telemedicine technologies, such as video conferencing with geographically distant colleagues, can help toward that goal, as can consulting the scientific literature, published ethics codes, and the "risk management" office within the clinical institution.

The fifth ethical skill is the ability to recognize high-risk situations that are more likely to give rise to ethical problems. Those often involve scenarios in which the healthcare professional has to step outside the familiar clinical role to take measures aimed at protecting the patient's interest (even if the patient disagrees) or a third party deemed in danger on the basis of information obtained during treatment. Involuntary treatment, where the patient refuses the recommended intervention but is deemed unable to provide informed consent, and emergency lifesaving treatment, where the informed consent process cannot be followed due to time restrictions or patient trauma, are two such scenarios. Consider the example of a woman with an intellectual disability who is in the third trimester of pregnancy and is brought to the emergency department by a roommate who noticed blood on the patient's clothing. The patient declines admission and asks to leave. This situation is high risk with respect to not only the pregnancy but also the physician's vulnerability to making ethical (and legal) mistakes. Stepping back to understand the situation clinically and legally, in accordance with ethical duties of the profession, will take careful consideration and, as described next, the laying in of appropriate safeguards for the patient.

Another example of a high-risk situation is one in which a physician has multiple or overlapping roles as both a clinical caregiver and a physician-scientist or as both a clinical caregiver and an administrator. Each professional role that a physician fulfills has a set of duties that may or may not neatly fit with those of other roles. A patient who is approached about entering a clinical trial may believe that his physician, who has always looked out for his best interest, will "sneak" the experimental medication to him, rather than honor the double-blind, placebo-controlled design. This phenomenon is referred to as the therapeutic misconception [43] and may be more likely when the caregiving physician also leads the research team, leaving the patient with the mistaken impression that *beneficence* rather than scientific integrity will govern his care.

The final skill deemed essential to ethical problem solving is the ability to build meaningful ethical safeguards into one's work. The intent of this skill is to create precautions that allow for better ethical decisions, in real time and in the future. Safeguards can work to prevent the emergence of new ethical problems as well. For example, pediatricians and other clinicians working with children should inform new patients and their families about the limits of *confidentiality* as they apply, among other mandates, to reporting child abuse. Similarly, researchers can avoid ethical conflicts by ensuring a well-trained research staff, encrypting data to protect subject information, developing user-friendly informed consent documents, allowing adequate time for questions during the consent process, and delineating an easy "exit" mechanism for volunteers wishing to withdraw from a study if they change their minds about participation.

Professionalism

Professionalism for physicians is intertwined with ethical responsibility and is hard to define independently. Professional skills can be thought about in three broad categories: interpersonal professionalism, public professionalism, and intrapersonal professionalism [44]. These rubrics are paired with key concepts (Table 1.3). It may be said

Table 1.3 Variations on a theme: three concepts of professionalism

Rubric	Key concepts
Interpersonal professionalism	Relationships and interactions with patients and colleagues
	Shared decision making
	Compassion
	Honesty
	Appropriate use of power
	Sensitivity to diverse populations
Public professionalism	Fulfilling the expectations society has for medical professionals
	Adherence to ethical codes
	Technical competency
	Enhancing the welfare of the community
Intrapersonal professionalism	Maintenance of the ability to function as a medical professional
	Self-awareness
	Knowledge of one's limits
	Lifelong learning
	Self-care

Reprinted with permission from Concise Guide to Ethics in Mental Health Care, (Copyright ©2004) and Professionalism and Ethics: Q & A Self-Study Guide for Mental Health Professionals (Copyright ©2008). American Psychiatric Association that professionalism "aspires to altruism, accountability, excellence, duty, service, honor, integrity, and respect for others" [45]. The American Board of Internal Medicine explains professionalism as "those skills, attitudes and behaviors which we have come to expect from individuals during the practice of their profession and includes concepts such as maintenance of competence, ethical behavior, integrity, honesty, altruism, service to others, adherence to professional codes, justice, respect for others, self-regulation, etc." [46]. The origins of many of these concepts are detailed in chapter "Professionalism in Medicine as a Transnational and Transcultural Ethical Concept". Some of the major themes of professionalism are highlighted in the following text.

Personal Responsibility

Incorporated into the idea of medical professionalism is a high standard of personal responsibility in areas that do not directly involve patient care. Most specialty boards require standards for off-the-clock behaviors for physicians and other healthcare professionals. For instance, there are expectations and codes against criminal behavior, excessive substance use, or conflicts of interest with regard to money matters or personal/sexual matters. These expectations may include issues of professional role like boundaries between doctors and patients, ensuring the least degree of personal interaction and the highest degree of professional (doctor/patient) interaction possible and appropriate. Licensing boards can and will take action against physicians' unprofessional behavior even when it is not directly related to their role in direct patient care.

Recognition and Resolution of Role Conflicts and Conflicts of Interest

Conflicts among various professional roles and related interests are an important area within professionalism. A physician's role in one aspect of professional life can create conflict in another. Physician relationships with for-profit companies such as the pharmaceutical industry, for example, can lead to professional pitfalls that can compromise the integrity of a physician's work [47]. Learning to identify and minimize the potential impact of role conflicts is an important developmental skill for physicians and physicians-in-training.

Recognizing and Addressing Issues Related to Impairment

The impaired physician is another example in which professional conduct and responsibility can be compromised. Physicians may be impaired as a result of substance use, disease, medication side effects, cognitive decline from advanced age or other etiologies, or other reasons. It is a professional responsibility to be aware of the level of one's performance and that of colleagues and to be alert to substance use or health and mental health issues that might impair it. Aiding the "impaired physician" and acting to rectify a situation if inappropriate and unprofessional behavior is suspected are professional duties [48].

Positive Duty to Engage in Lifelong Learning and Continued Education

Another professional value is dedication to continued education. Lifelong learning is a crucial activity for the medical professional. But the abilities to understand one's limits and make appropriate referral and/or gain appropriate consultation are also professional virtues. Growing one's medical knowledge and recognizing the limits of one's clinical scope and abilities are professional goals for every physician [49].

Teaching Biomedical Ethics

Over the last 25 years, the medical profession has steadily shifted from the view that ethics are not teachable to adopting educational curricula that systematically introduce students, trainees, and researchers to bioethical principles and their application. Several factors are propelling this shift: the need to recapture the moral stature historically accorded to healthcare professionals, the empowerment of patients in clinical decision-making, rapid changes in healthcare methods and systems, and the changing demographic and cultural mosaic within which healthcare delivery occurs. Other likely contributing factors include limited resources and seemingly unlimited demand, the medicolegal complexities of current medical practice, the information technology revolution and its effects on medicine, and the growing desire by medical professionals to balance busy healthcare careers with personal time. These changes have brought new ethical challenges that, absent solid foundation in bioethics, can be disorienting and difficult to respond to – hence, the expanding attempts to disseminate and teach bioethics. Chapter "Ethical Issues in Biomedical Research and Clinical Training" outlines many of the cardinal ethical issues experienced in clinical training.

The Liaison Committee on Medical Education, the accrediting authority for medical schools in the United States and Canada, counts the following criterion among its accreditation standards [50]: "A medical school must teach medical ethics and human values, and require its students to exhibit scrupulous ethical principles in caring for patients, and in relating to patients' families and to others involved in patient care." Similarly, the Accreditation Council for Graduate Medical Education, which oversees residency training programs, requires the teaching and demonstration of general competencies in ethics as a requirement for accreditation and specialty certification [51].

As further examples, the American Board of Pediatrics and the American Board of Internal Medicine have required formal ethics education and tested competency in their certifying examinations, since the mid-1980s. These boards have emphasized how the goal of an ethics education is not to teach for an examination but to teach lifelong skills in a manner that is attuned to the ecology of clinical practice. Innovative performance-based approaches to evaluating ethical skills have been developed, for example, having a trained professional observe an early-career physician obtain informed consent or refusal for an intervention from an ambivalent patient – and doing so in a manner that truly informs, does not coerce, and does foster authentic decision-making. It is anticipated that these methods of evaluating physician skill will be widely adopted in time, as will other efforts to integrate quality measures, patient satisfaction measures, and ethical standards in clinical care practice.

Conclusion

We have presented key definitions and concepts in bioethics along with how they might translate in clinical and research contexts, arguing that biomedical ethics is a "living" scholarly discipline of which systematic application and teaching strengthen the healthcare profession. The value of ethically informed decision-making is readily apparent in high-stake clinical and biomedical research situations, but every-day clinical practice, investigation, and training bring a multitude of smaller decisions and actions, each filled with ethical meaning. With every patient seen, research protocol designed, prescription written, and piece of medical advice offered, there is an opportunity to embody ancient but highly relevant ethical principles in a manner that reaffirms their centrality to modern medicine and professionalism.

Review and Reflect: Ask Yourself and Talk with Colleagues

For each of the following scenarios, ask yourself and talk with colleagues about the following questions: What ethical tensions exist in this situation? How can the physician or physician-in-training in this scenario apply fundamental ethics "skills" and fulfill obligations of professionalism?

Scenario 1 For 9 months, a primary care provider in a rural environment has treated a woman whose spouse is in the military and has been deployed to the Middle East for the past 6 months. A week after the patient's last visit to the provider, the two encountered each other at the local grocery store, and the patient introduced the physician to her family. During the discussion, the physician learned that he and the patient's father have a mutual interest in hunting, and the family subsequently invited him to join them for dinner at the restaurant next to the store. Later that week, the physician is processing a specialty consult for the patient. He calls to let her know that she needs to complete some additional paperwork. The patient notes that her parents are visiting and invites the physician to come to dinner and bring the paperwork with him.

Scenario 2 A 49-year-old patient asks a sports medicine physician to provide treatment that lacks data but has developed celebrity cache: platelet-rich plasma for sports injuries. The patient is an accomplished body builder who acknowledges that he has taken testosterone supplements in the past, although has never used illicit substances or steroids ("those things are bad for you, right? Testosterone is 'natural' – a little more doesn't hurt"). The patient spends most of his nonwork time in sports activities and recently has taken up mixed martial arts.

Scenario 3 A resident physician in a teaching hospital speaks with a patient who seems to understand fully the risks and benefits of a proposed medication. The patient is willing to begin the new treatment. The resident notes that the patient has a legal guardian, however, and is not sure about how to approach informed consent in this context because the patient appears capable of making the decision and "is agreeable."

Scenario 4 On the obstetric labor floor, fetal distress is detected and the resident attempts to counsel the patient that Cesarean section is recommended by the attending physician. The patient and her husband decline the Cesarean section because of their "cultural" beliefs, offering no other explanation. Half an hour passes. The attending and the chief resident counsel the patient, recommending Cesarean section again, given continued distressed status of the fetus. The patient verbally consents; however, her husband declines and accuses the doctors of wanting to do a Cesarean section because "that is what makes the most money for the hospital."

Scenario 5 A female adolescent with anorexia nervosa is admitted to the adolescent medicine ward for low body weight and refusal to eat. She tells the pediatrician that only smoking marijuana allows her to eat. They agree that she will take a blinded regimen that may contain a cannabis derivative, and the patient resumes eating and gaining weight. The patient begins telling other patients on the unit that her pediatrician is giving her marijuana and she is getting much better because of it. One of these patients with a diagnosis of major depression and low appetite approaches the pediatrician and asks for the same regimen in order to improve his low body weight. He insists that he be treated the same as the other patients on the ward.

Scenario 6 A 16-year-old young woman presents for a routine wellness physical examination. When the clinician asks if she has ever experienced abuse, she responds, "Are you going to tell anybody? I will only talk to you about it if you promise not to." The clinician fears that if he tells the patient he is legally required to report child abuse, she may not confide in him and he might miss an opportunity to help her. He also knows that if she does confide in him about potential abuse, he will have to break confidentiality and report this abuse to law enforcement, which may alienate her.

Scenario 7 A 36-year-old male patient who travels internationally 60 % of the year describes to his primary care physician a 6-month history of difficulty with fatigue, wakefulness, concentration, and memory, and he attributes his difficulty to frequent changes in time zone. The man denies symptoms consistent with sleep apnea or narcolepsy and does not perform shift work. He asks for a prescription of a stimulant to "get back up to speed and be on my toes." He has no active health problems or personal or family history of heart disease or sudden death. Because his use of the medication would be off-label and he is not suffering with significant clinical impairment, the physician is unsure whether to prescribe this medication.

Scenario 8 A civilian primary care physician works in a military hospital, caring for service members in a specialized unit for wounded service members that is focused toward rehabilitation, recovery, and transition back to duty or out of the military. As part of the management of a particular patient, the physician orders routine urine drug screens to ensure compliance with their sole provider agreement and medication regimen. The patient reports that he continues to take oxycodone on an as-needed basis (4–6 tablets per week) and has continued to get prescriptions. On one of the routine urine drug screens, the physician finds that the patient's urine is negative for any oxycodone but is positive for hydrocodone.

Scenario 9 A 20-year-old woman has undergone extensive work-up for seizures, which video EEG has found to be psychogenic seizures. During another episode overnight, a resident asks the nurse to administer normal saline through the IV and to tell the patient, "This is something that might make you feel better." The patient's episode stops shortly thereafter. The resident suggests at morning rounds that giving IV saline during psychogenic episodes becomes part of the treatment plan for this patient. The resident wonders whether giving placebo as part of this patient's treatment plan would be ethical.

Acknowledgments The following authors contributed to the scenarios in this chapter: Laura Weiss Roberts, M.D., M.A., Daryn Reicherter, M.D., Richard Balon, M.D., Jodi K. Casados, M.D., Kristi R. Estabrook, M.D., Michelle Goldsmith, M.D., M.A., Celeste Lopez, M.D., Christine Moutier, M.D., Richard Shaw, M.D., Christopher Warner, M.D., LTC.

References

1. Gray FD. The Tuskegee Syphilis Study. Montgomery: Black Belt Press; 1998.
2. Advisory Committee on Human Radiation Experiments. The human radiation experiments. New York: Oxford University Press; 1996.
3. Beecher HK. Ethics and clinical research. N Engl J Med. 1966;274:1354–60.
4. O'Donnell JJ. Cassiodorus. Berkeley: University of California Press; 1969.

5. American Medical Association. Garrison & Morton, Medical Bib., 5th ed, 1764; Pellegrino, "Thomas Percival's Ethics" Introduction to Medical ethics, Classics of Med. Lib. Spec. Ed.
6. Aksoy S. The religious tradition of Ishaq ibn Ali al-Ruhawi: the author of the first medical ethics book in Islamic medicine. J Int Soc Hist Islamic Med. 2004;3:9–11.
7. Lasagna L. "Hippocratic Oath—Modern Version". WGBH Educational Foundation for PBS and NOVA Online. 1964. ethics.ucsd.edu/journal/2006/readings/Hippocratic_Oath_Modern_Version.pdf. Accessed 12 May 2014.
8. American Medical Association. Principles of medical ethics. 2001. http://www.ama-assn.org/ama/pub/physician-resources/medical-ethics/code-medical-ethics/principles-medical-ethics.page?. Accessed 30 Apr 2014.
9. American Medical Association. History of medical ethics. 2001. http://www.ama-assn.org/ama/pub/physician-resources/medical-ethics/code-medical-ethics/history-ama-ethics.page. Accessed 21 Jan 2012.
10. Project of the ABIM Foundation, ACP–ASIM Foundation, European Federation of Internal Medicine. Medical professionalism in the new millennium: a physician charter. Ann Int Med. 2002;136(3):243–6.
11. American Board of Pediatrics. Bioethics. 2001. https://www.abp.org/abpwebsite/publicat/bioethics.pdf. Accessed 30 Jan 2012.
12. American College of Physicians. Ethics issues. 2012. http://www.acponline.org/running_practice/ethics/issues. Accessed 30 Jan 2012.
13. American Psychiatric Association. Ethics. 2010. http://www.psych.org/MainMenu/PsychiatricPractice/Ethics.aspx. Accessed 21 Jan 2012.
14. American College of Surgeons. Code of professional conduct. 2003. http://www.facs.org/memberservices/codeofconduct.html. Accessed 21 Jan 2012.
15. The American Heart Association. Code of ethics. 2010. http://www.heart.org/HEARTORG/General/American-Heart-Association-Ethics-Policy-Details_UCM_300431_Article.jsp#.TyYr5_mwUgo. Accessed 29 Jan 2012.
16. The College of American Pathologists. Code of ethics. 2009. http://www.cap.org/apps/cap.portal?_nfpb=true&cntvwrPtlt_actionOverride=%2Fportlets%2FcontentViewer%2Fshow&_windowLabel=cntvwrPtlt&cntvwrPtlt{actionForm.contentReference}=cap_foundation%2FCode_of_Ethics.html&_state=maximized&_pageLabel=cntvwr. Accessed 30 Jan 2012.
17. The American Academy of Dermatology. Code of medical ethics for dermatologists. 2011. http://www.aad.org/Forms/Policies/Uploads/AR/AR%20Code%20of%20Medical%20Ethics%20for%20Dermatologists.pdf. Accessed 29 Jan 2012.
18. American Psychological Association. Ethical principles of psychologists and code of conduct. 2010. http://www.apa.org/ethics/code/index.aspx. Accessed 21 Jan 2012.
19. American Pharmacists Association. Code of ethics for pharmacists. 1994. http://www.pharmacist.com/AM/Template.cfm?Section=Search1&template=/CM/HTMLDisplay.cfm&ContentID=2903. Accessed 29 Jan 2012.
20. American Nurses Association. Code of ethics for nurses. http://nursingworld.org/MainMenuCategories/ThePracticeofProfessionalNursing/EthicsStandards/CodeofEthics.aspx. Accessed 21 Jan 2012.
21. National Association of Social Workers. Code of ethics, 2008. http://www.socialworkers.org/pubs/code/default.asp. Accessed 29 Jan 2012.
22. Annas GJ, Grodin MA, editors. The Nazi doctors and the nuremberg code: human rights in human experimentation. New York: Oxford University Press; 1992.
23. World Medical Association. Declaration of Helsinki. 2008. http://www.wma.net/en/20activities/10ethics/10helsinki/index.html. Accessed 21 Jan 2012.
24. National Institutes of Health. The Belmont report. 1979. http://ohsr.od.nih.gov/guidelines/belmont.html. Accessed 21 Jan 2012.
25. Russell, WMS, Burch, RL. The principles of humane experimental technique. 1959. http://altweb.jhsph.edu/pubs/books/humane_exp/het-toc. Accessed 27 May 2014.
26. Festing S, Wilkinson R. The ethics of animal research. EMBO Rep. 2007;8(6):526–30.

27. American Psychological Association. Guidelines for ethical conduct in the care and use of animals. http://www.apa.org/science/leadership/care/guidelines.aspx. Accessed 21 Jan 2012.
28. Aboujaoude E. Ethics commentary: ethical challenges in the treatment of anxiety. Focus. 2011;9:289–91.
29. Roberts LW, Dyer A. A concise guide to ethics in mental health care. Washington, DC: American Psychiatric Publishing; 2004.
30. Grisso T, Appelbaum PS. The MacArthur competence study, III: abilities of patients to consent to psychiatric and medical treatments. Law Hum Behav. 1995;19:149–74.
31. Grisso T, Appelbaum PS, Mulvey EP, et al. The MacArthur Competence Study, II: abilities of patients to consent to psychiatric and medical treatments. Law Hum Behav. 1995;19:127–48.
32. Appelbaum PS, Grisso T. The MacArthur Competence Study, I: mental illness and competence to consent to treatment. Law Hum Behav. 1995;19:105–26.
33. Lundberg GD. Severed trust. New York: Basic Books; 2002.
34. Institute of Medicine: Preserving Public Trust. Accreditation and human research participant protection programs. Washington, DC: National Academy Press; 2001.
35. Williams CT, Fost N. Ethical considerations surrounding first time procedures: a study and analysis of patient attitudes toward spinal taps by students. Kennedy Inst Ethics J. 1992;2(3):217.
36. Department of Health and Human Services. Obama administration issues rules requiring parity in treatment of mental, substance use disorders. 2010. http://www.hhs.gov/news/press/2010pres/01/20100129a.html. Accessed 1 Feb 2012.
37. Groves JE. Taking care of the hateful patient. N Engl J Med. 1978;298(16):883–7.
38. McCarty T, Roberts LW. The difficult patient. In: Rubin RH, Voss C, Derksen D, Gateley A, Quenzer R, editors. Medicine: a primary care approach. Philadelphia: WB Saunders; 1996. p. 395–9.
39. Lloyd, GER editor. Hippocratic writings. Translated by Chadwick, J, Mann, WN. Harmondsworth: Penguin; 1978.
40. Tarasoff v Regents of the University of California, 17 Cal.3d 425;551 P.2d 334 (Cal. Rptr. 14, 1976)
41. US Department of Health and Human Services. The Health Insurance Portability and Accountability Act (HIPAA) of 1996. http://www.hhs.gov/ocr/privacy/. Accessed 11 May 2014.
42. Gelso CJ, Hayes JA. Counter transference and the therapist's inner experience: perils and possibilities. Mahwah: Lawrence Erlbaum Associates; 2007. p. 59.
43. Lidz CW, Appelbaum PS. The therapeutic misconception: problems and solutions. Med Care. 2002;40(9 Suppl):55–63.
44. Roberts LW, Hoop JG. Professionalism and ethics: Q&A self-study guide for mental health professionals. Washington, DC: American Psychiatric Publishing; 2008.
45. Canadian Medical Association. Series of health care discussion papers: professionalism in medicine. Ottawa: Canadian Medical Association; 2001.
46. American Board of Internal Medicine. Medical professionalism in the new millennium: a physician charter. 2004.
47. American Medical Association. Opinion 8.03 – Conflicts of interest: guidelines issued July 1986; Updated June 1994.
48. American Medical Association. Opinion 9.031 – Reporting Impaired, Incompetent, or Unethical Colleagues, adopted Dec 2003.
49. Association of American Medical Colleges, American Association of Colleges of Nursing. Lifelong learning in medicine and nursing: final conference report. 2010. http://www.aacn.nche.edu/education-resources/MacyReport.pdf. Accessed 31 Mar 2014.
50. Liaison Committee on Medical Education. Accreditation Standard ED-23. http://www.iaomc.org/lcme.htm
51. Accreditation Council for Graduate Medical Education. Institutional requirements. 2003. http://www.acgme.org/acWebsite/irc/irc_IRCpr703.asp#IA. Accessed 21 Jan 2012.

Recommended Reading

American Medical Association Council on Ethical and Judicial Affairs: Code of Medical Ethics, Current Opinions with Annotations. Available at http://www.ama-assn.org/ama/pub/physician-resources/medical-ethics/code-medical-ethics.page. Accessed 29 May 2014.

American Medical Association: Code of Medical Ethics 2012–2013 Current Opinions With Annotations. Chicago: American Medical Association; 2012.

Junkerman C, Schiedermayer D. Practical ethics for students, interns and residents. A short reference manual. 2nd ed. Frederick: University Publishing Group; 1998.

Reynolds R, Stone J, editors. On doctoring. 3rd ed. New York: Free Press; 2001.

Chapter 2
The Legal Framework of Medical Ethics in the United States

Joseph B. Layde

Medical ethical principles are supported by a legal framework. In the United States, a body of law arising from judicial opinions, statutes, and administrative rulings constitutes an important background for an overview of medical ethics in a book such as this one. This chapter provides an overview of the legal foundation of medical ethics likely to be of interest to the student and practitioner.

Each of the 50 states of the United States is its own jurisdiction; the federal government constitutes a 51st jurisdiction. The Supremacy Clause of the US Constitution states that federal law trumps state law, but there are many areas of medical ethics in which there is no federal law or controlling federal judicial ruling. In addition, judicial opinions sometimes change over time. In short, the following selected legal cases and legislative actions are intended to show a range of legal approaches to common problems in medical ethics.

The cases, statutes, and rules described in this chapter are grouped in several general areas of medical ethical interest. Many of the entries involve several ethical principles and highlight the tension between them. Courts and legislatures grant considerable deference to personal autonomy, for instance, but that deference is not absolute. It is hoped that these materials will lead the reader to appreciate the struggle the legal system shares with medicine in determining what right or principle trumps another in a given medical ethical dilemma.

Sources of medical-legal frameworks in US law are established through different mechanisms and provide different expectations in different jurisdictions. Major sources of US law are summarized in Table 2.1.

J.B. Layde, M.D., J.D. (✉)
Department of Psychiatry and Behavioral Medicine, Medical College of Wisconsin,
Milwaukee, WI, USA
e-mail: jlayde@mcw.edu

© Springer Science+Business Media New York 2015

L.W. Roberts, D. Reicherter (eds.), *Professionalism and Ethics in Medicine*,
DOI 10.1007/978-1-4939-1686-3_2

Table 2.1 Sources of law

US constitution	Provides basic structure of federal government and (with amendments including Bill of Rights) outlines individual protections. Includes Supremacy Clause, which determines that valid federal law trumps state law in case of conflict
State constitutions	Provide basic structure of each state government and include individual protections—may be more explicit than Bill of Rights—e.g., may include specifically listed right to privacy
Federal statutes	Enacted by US Congress; may apply to entire nation
State statutes	Enacted by state legislatures; apply to individual state
Federal regulations	Enacted by executive branch of US government to give specificity to federal legislative enactments; may apply to entire nation
State regulations	Enacted by executive branch of state government to give specificity to state legislative enactments; apply to individual state
Federal judicial decisions	Clarify uncertain areas of federal law; may determine whether federal statute or state constitution or statute violates US Constitution; US Supreme Court decisions may apply to entire nation
State judicial decisions	Clarify uncertain areas of state law; apply to individual state

Cases, Statutes, and Rules

Decision-Making by Competent Patients

Schloendorff v. Society of New York Hospital

Mary E. Schloendorff was suffering from what the Court of Appeals of New York (the highest court in the state) called "some disorder of the stomach" [1]. She agreed to be treated at the New York Hospital (for $7 per week) and to undergo an ether examination to determine the nature of a fibroid tumor and allegedly stipulated, "There must be no operation" to remove the tumor. While she was unconscious from the ether, she said, the tumor was removed without her knowledge or consent. In his opinion, Judge Benjamin Cardozo wrote:

> In the case at hand, the wrong complained of is not merely negligence. It is trespass. Every human being of adult years and sound mind has a right to determine what shall be done with his own body; and a surgeon who performs an operation without his patient's consent, commits an assault for which he is liable in damages.

The court held, however, that the nonprofit New York Hospital was not responsible for the actions of the doctors and nurses in the case and that the patient was not entitled to damages from the hospital.

The language by Judge Cardozo in this case sets the framework for the primacy of autonomy in medical ethics in the United States. It is important to note that he limited his endorsement of patient autonomy in medical decision-making to competent adults. This case is one of the most frequently cited cases in medical ethics literature.

Application of President and Directors of Georgetown College

Jesse E. Jones, an adult woman suffering from a ruptured ulcer who was a Jehovah's Witness, refused on religious grounds to receive blood transfusions that her doctors felt were necessary to save her life. Her husband (also a Jehovah's Witness) refused to intervene, and Georgetown University Hospital sought permission to give her the transfusions involuntarily [2]. The patient was the mother of a 7-month-old child. The Federal District Court in the District of Columbia refused to authorize transfusions, but a Court of Appeals judge signed an order permitting "such transfusions to Mrs. Jones as might be 'necessary to save her life.'"

This case is an interesting outlier and points out the willingness of some courts (at least historically) to allow exceptions to the general rule of patient autonomy in medical decision-making in situations in which there are particular exigencies, such as the existence of a young child who would lose a parent in an emergent medical situation if a contemplated treatment that is refused by the patient is not given.

Decision-Making for Incompetent Patients

Strunk v. Strunk

The mother and "committee" (guardian) of Jerry Strunk, an incompetent 27-year-old man with severe intellectual disability, petitioned a Kentucky court for permission to authorize the transplant of one of Jerry Strunk's kidneys into his brother Tommy Strunk, a 28-year-old part-time college student who suffered from chronic glomerulonephritis [3]. The case was heard by the Court of Appeals of Kentucky (which was at the time the highest court in the state), which authorized the transplant, finding that donating the kidney to his brother was in the best interest of Jerry Strunk. The court believed that giving his brother the chance to live would benefit Jerry, given the close tie he felt with his brother Tommy.

In re Quinlan

Karen Ann Quinlan entered a persistent vegetative state after a period of anoxia. She was maintained on life support, including a mechanical ventilator [4]. She was not brain dead, but her father, applying to act as her guardian, asked to have her ventilator removed. There was little evidence as to what the patient would have wanted done had she been able to decide for herself what care to receive. The Supreme Court of New Jersey, citing the privacy rights of the incompetent patient and the desire of her father to exercise what he believed to be the proper substituted judgment as to what she would have wanted done, decided the following:

> Upon the concurrence of the guardian and family of Karen, should the responsible attending physicians conclude that there is no reasonable possibility of Karen's ever emerging from her present comatose condition to a cognitive, sapient state and that the life-support apparatus now being administered to Karen should be discontinued, they shall consult with the hospital "Ethics Committee" or like body of the institution in which Karen is then hospitalized. If that consultative body agrees that there is no reasonable possibility of Karen's ever emerging from her present comatose condition to a cognitive, sapient state, the present life-support system may be withdrawn and said action shall be without any civil or criminal liability therefore on the part of any participant, whether guardian, physician, hospital or others.

Superintendent of Belchertown State School and Another v. Joseph Saikewicz

Joseph Saikewicz, an incompetent 67-year-old man with severe intellectual disability, suffered from acute myeloblastic monocytic leukemia [5]. The Supreme Judicial Court of Massachusetts (the highest court in the state) upheld a probate judge's ruling that chemotherapy not be administered to the incompetent patient. The court held that the proper rule for consenting to or declining medical treatment for an incompetent person was that of substituted judgment, in which the decision-maker attempts to apply the wishes of the incompetent person. Mr. Saikewicz had never been competent, so he had never had the chance to enunciate his wishes regarding medical treatment. The court wrote that that the probate judge had properly relied in declining the treatment for him, in part, on the fact that Mr. Saikewicz was incapable of fully understanding the purpose of intrusive chemotherapy but would nevertheless suffer from the side effects of such chemotherapy.

Interestingly, by the time the Supreme Judicial Court of Massachusetts issued its opinion in the case, Joseph Saikewicz had already died of bronchial pneumonia as a complication of his leukemia.

Cruzan by Cruzan v. Director, Missouri Department of Health

Nancy Cruzan was a young woman who was rendered incompetent when she was in a severe car crash in Missouri [6, 7]. She was in a persistent vegetative state when her parents asked to have her artificial nutrition and hydration stopped, citing Nancy's conversation with a housemate before her accident, in which she had said that she would not want to continue life if she could not live at least somewhat normally. The US Supreme Court upheld the Supreme Court of Missouri's right to require "clear and convincing evidence" of Nancy's desire to have life-sustaining treatment discontinued in order for her treatment to be stopped.

Eventually, Nancy Cruzan's parents were able to present sufficient evidence of Nancy's wishes to meet the "clear and convincing evidence" standard required by the Missouri courts, and she died after her life-sustaining measures were stopped.

Patient Self-Determination Act of 1990

The US Congress, taking up issues raised in the *Cruzan* case as it made its way up the ladder of appellate review, mandated that hospitals, nursing facilities, home health agencies, hospice programs, and health maintenance organizations receiving federal funding inform patients of their right to make advance directives to appoint healthcare agents or to write living wills [8].

Rights of Infants – "Baby Doe Rules"

Following a series of controversies, including one involving "Baby Doe," an infant born in Bloomington, Indiana, with Down syndrome and esophageal atresia with tracheoesophageal fistula who died after the parents declined to authorize corrective surgery, the US Congress passed legislation in 1984 authorizing the Department of Health and Human Services to write federal regulations intended to safeguard the rights of handicapped infants [9, 10]. The rules continue to be in force to prevent child abuse, although a number of legal challenges have limited the ways the federal government can enforce them.

The current rules call for a notice such as the following to be posted at federally funded healthcare agencies caring for infants:

Principles of Treatment of Disabled Infants

It is the policy of this hospital, consistent with Federal law, that nourishment and medically beneficial treatment (as determined with respect for reasonable medical judgments) should not be withheld from handicapped infants solely on the basis of their present or anticipated mental or physical impairments.

The rules go on to give guidance on the care of handicapped infants as follows (including the first paragraph below), quoting the "Principles of Treatment of Disabled Infants" promulgated by a coalition of organizations, including the American Academy of Pediatrics and the Association for Retarded Citizens:

When medical care is clearly beneficial, it should always be provided. When appropriate medical care is not available, arrangements should be made to transfer the infant to an appropriate medical facility. Consideration such as anticipated or actual limited potential of an individual and present or future lack of available community resources are irrelevant and must not determine the decisions concerning medical care. The individual's medical condition should be the sole focus of the decision. These are very strict standards.

It is ethically and legally justified to withhold medical or surgical procedures which are clearly futile and will only prolong the act of dying. However, supportive care should be provided, including sustenance as medically indicated and relief of pain and suffering. The needs of the dying person should be respected. The family also should be supported in its grieving.

In cases where it is uncertain whether medical treatment will be beneficial, a person's disability must not be the basis for a decision to withhold treatment. At all times during the process when decisions are being made about the benefit or futility of medical treatment, the person should be cared for in the medically most appropriate ways. When doubt exists at any time about whether to treat, a presumption always should be in favor of treatment.

Ethics of Reproductive Health

Griswold v. Connecticut

The US Supreme Court considered a case in which the executive director of Planned Parenthood of Connecticut and a Yale Medical School professor challenged a Connecticut statute under which they were arrested in 1961 for providing contraception (to married persons!) and eventually found guilty [11]. The majority opinion in the case, written by Justice William Douglas, invalidated the Connecticut statute on the grounds that it violated a right to privacy which the court found was protected by the "penumbra" of specifically delineated guarantees in the Bill of Rights. Justice Douglas wrote:

> The present case, then, concerns a relationship lying within the zone of privacy created by several fundamental constitutional guarantees. And it concerns a law which, in forbidding the use of contraceptives, rather than regulating their manufacture or sale, seeks to achieve its goals by means having a maximum destructive impact upon that relationship. Such a law cannot stand in light of the familiar principle, so often applied by this Court, that a governmental purpose to control or prevent activities constitutionally subject to state regulation may not be achieved by means which sweep unnecessarily broadly and thereby invade the area of protected freedoms.
> NAACP v. Alabama, 377 U.S. 288, 307. Would we allow the police to search the sacred precincts of marital bedrooms for telltale signs of the use of contraceptives? The [p486] very idea is repulsive to the notions of privacy surrounding the marriage relationship.
> We deal with a right of privacy older than the Bill of Rights – older than our political parties, older than our school system. Marriage is a coming together for better or for worse, hopefully enduring, and intimate to the degree of being sacred. It is an association that promotes a way of life, not causes; a harmony in living, not political faiths; a bilateral loyalty, not commercial or social projects. Yet it is an association for as noble a purpose as any involved in our prior decisions.

This landmark case identified the constitutionally protected right to privacy that has been the basis for many other medical cases since 1964, including the 1973 case of Roe v. Wade [12]. In light of current views in society, it is remarkable that a physician could be convicted in Connecticut for prescribing contraceptives—the case illustrates the relatively recent legal recognition of a medical right to privacy which we now take for granted.

Roe v. Wade

The US Supreme Court considered the constitutionality of the Texas statute criminalizing abortion, and in one of the most famous and controversial US Supreme Court opinions in history, Justice Blackmun wrote the majority opinion, striking down the law as a violation of the right to privacy contained in the penumbra of the Bill of Rights [12].

A single woman from Texas using the pseudonym Jane Roe found in 1970 that she was unable to obtain a legal abortion in Texas. She sued to overturn the Texas law that prohibited her from obtaining one, and the US Supreme Court held that because the normal length of a pregnancy is shorter than the length of the typical legal appellate process, the case was not "moot" (i.e., there was still an active controversy about the case) when it addressed the issues raised by her suit years later. The majority opinion ruled that the constitutionally protected right to privacy forbids a state from criminalizing abortion early in pregnancy. States are permitted increasing discretion in regulating abortions later in the course of pregnancy and may criminalize it after the stage of pregnancy at which the fetus becomes viable, except in cases in which abortion is necessary to preserve the life or health of the mother.

Hastening the End of Life

Oregon Death with Dignity Act

The voters of Oregon passed a ballot initiative in 1994 permitting physician-assisted suicide in the state [13]. After a series of challenges, the Death with Dignity Act became law in Oregon in 1997, making Oregon the first US jurisdiction to allow physician-assisted suicide. It makes the following provision:

> An adult who is capable, is a resident of Oregon, and has been determined by the attending physician and consulting physician to be suffering from a terminal disease, and who has voluntarily expressed his or her wish to die, may make a written request for medication for the purpose of ending his or her life in a humane and dignified manner in accordance with ORS 127.800 to 127.897.

Psychiatric Treatment

Lessard v. Schmidt

Alberta Lessard, a Wisconsin schoolteacher, challenged the state's civil commitment law under which she had been detained, alleging that the statute denied her due process of law in permitting her detention up to 145 days without a hearing, in failing to give a right to counsel at a reasonable time, in allowing hearsay evidence in proceedings, and on other grounds [14]. A three-judge panel of federal judges in Milwaukee agreed with her in most respects and stated:

> We conclude that the Wisconsin civil commitment procedure is constitutionally defective insofar as it fails to require effective and timely notice of the "charges" under which a person is sought to be detained; fails to require adequate notice of all rights, including the

right to jury trial; permits detention longer than 48 hours without a hearing on probable cause; permits detention longer than two weeks without a full hearing on the necessity for commitment; permits commitment based upon a hearing in which the person charged with mental illness is not represented by adversary counsel, at which hearsay evidence is admitted, and in which psychiatric evidence is presented without the patient having been given the benefit of the privilege against self-incrimination; permits commitment without proof beyond a reasonable doubt that the patient is both "mentally ill" and dangerous; and fails to require those seeking commitment to consider less restrictive alternatives to commitment.

The court's judgment in the *Lessard v. Schmidt* became the basis for Wisconsin's revised civil commitment statute and was very influential in other jurisdictions as well. The requirement of proof beyond a reasonable doubt was later changed to a requirement of proof by clear and convincing evidence after the US Supreme Court permitted that standard in *Addington v. Texas* [15]. *Lessard v. Schmidt* set the tone for heightened skepticism of laws mandating coerced psychiatric treatment in the years since it was decided; the opinion has been criticized for "criminalizing" procedures for civil commitment, even using the term "charges" (quotes in original) to describe the allegations leading to civil commitment proceedings.

Vitaly Tarasoff et al. v. The Regents of the University of California

Pronsenjit Poddar, a student at the University of California Berkeley, told his mental health caregivers at the student health center there that he planned to kill Berkeley resident Tatiana Tarasoff, who had not requited his love for her. The student health center did not take sufficient action to protect Ms. Tarasoff, and Poddar did in fact kill her. Her family sued the university.

The Supreme Court of California issued two opinions in the case [16, 17]—in 1974, the court found there was a "duty to warn" identifiable likely victims of violent mental health outpatients. On reconsideration of the case in 1976 after much controversy and confusion arose from its 1974 decision, the court refined its opinion to state that there is a "duty to protect" identifiable likely victims of reasonably foreseeable violence perpetrated by mental health outpatients in California, which might be fulfilled by warning the victim or by ensuring adequate secure treatment of the likely violent patient. Many other jurisdictions have followed or refined the California rule set in this very influential decision, which summarized its limitation to patient confidentiality as follows:

> We conclude that the public policy favoring protection of the confidential character of patient-psychotherapist communications must yield to the extent to which disclosure is essential to avert danger to others. The protective privilege ends where the public peril begins.

Confidentiality

Rule on Confidentiality of Alcohol and Drug Abuse Treatment Records

Health Insurance Portability and Accountability Act of 1996

The US Congress mandated in the 1996 Health Insurance Portability and Accountability Act (HIPAA) that the Department of Health and Human Services formulate privacy and security rules for protected health information [18–20]. The rules took effect over a graduated period from 2003 to 2006 and provide a layer of federal protection to the confidentiality of protected health information and emphasized the importance of security in the electronic transmission of health records. HIPAA rules extend federal confidentiality protection to patients receiving healthcare in general; the previously enacted Rule on Confidentiality of Alcohol and Drug Abuse Treatment Records continues to provide special protection to those patients receiving care for substance use disorders. Release of information forms often provide special checkmarks so that patients can indicate if they wish their substance use disorder treatment records, protected under 42 CFR Part 2, to be included in materials released by a healthcare agency.

Conclusion

The judicial opinions and legislative actions described in this chapter comprise some of the most important and interesting responses of the US legal system to the problems physicians and other healthcare workers face in grappling with difficult clinical situations that involve the need to respect persons, to do what is helpful and to avoid doing harm, and to attempt to do so in a just manner. The questions and answers that constitute the bulk of this book explore the application of these ethical principles in a wider variety of clinical contexts; the legal framework of bioethics gives some guidance but does not give all the answers to medical ethical dilemmas.

Review and Reflect: Ask Yourself and Talk with Colleagues

For each of the following scenarios, ask yourself and talk with colleagues about the following questions: What ethical tensions exist in this situation? What legal obligations, if any, are present? What are the clinician's next steps?

Scenario 1 A family practice physician provides prenatal care for a woman until her 36th week of pregnancy, at which time she transfers to the obstetrician who will facilitate her delivery. The woman returns to the family physician's office 2 weeks later, stating that she has not felt the baby move for 2 days. She told the obstetrician her concerns the day before, and he assured her once he auscultated fetal heart tones with the Doppler. The woman still felt worried, however. Upon further investigation, the family physician notes that she has suffered an intrauterine fetal demise. The physician is troubled, because the standard practice is to obtain a nonstress test in a patient with a 38-week gestation who complains of decreased fetal movement, and wonders why the obstetrician did not do this test. The test may have indicated fetal distress, at which time delivery or a Cesarean section could have been performed.

Scenario 2 A psychiatrist member of a medical school's committee on rank and tenure is reviewing materials from applicants for promotion in various departments of the school in advance of a committee meeting. He reads the promotion packet for a seemingly well-qualified assistant professor of dermatology who is applying for promotion to the rank of associate professor. The psychiatrist has treated the dermatologist for cannabis abuse and depression but believes that he is doing well currently.

Scenario 3 The sister-in-law of a physician's friend has severe fibromyalgia, which was previously treated very successfully with a novel medication. Unfortunately, she has lost her job, no longer has insurance, and cannot afford the medication. The physician's friend has a job with great benefits and asks the physician if he would prescribe the medication in the friend's name so that he might obtain it under his prescription plan and then give it to his wife.

Scenario 4 A primary care provider treats a 26-year-old man who uses crystal methamphetamine on the weekends and has unprotected sexual intercourse. He is planning a trip to a gay resort and has already obtained methamphetamine for his stay there. The physician worries about how to provide optimal care to this patient.

Scenario 5 A nursing home sends an elderly, wheelchair-bound man who has had a stroke to the hospital because he continually calls the police, saying that Jesus has told him the nursing staff are abusing him. In the hospital, the patient shares a room with a high-functioning man recovering from an orthopedic injury. The following day the elderly patient tells the attending physician that the hospital nursing staff ignore his requests for help to use the bathroom and so he has soiled himself. His roommate confirms his story and adds that he has been helping the patient use the bathroom as a result. The roommate, who is being discharged, is concerned for the elderly man's safety.

Scenario 6 A very helpful colleague asks a physician to write a letter supporting his application for clinical privileges that the physician feels are beyond the scope of his training.

Scenario 7 A 45-year-old diabetic man obtains medical care in a multidisciplinary clinic. He sees one doctor for primary care issues and another for psychiatric issues.

He has been living with diabetes for 20 years and has struggled with diabetic neuropathy in the past. As a result, he takes high doses of pain medications, prescribed by the primary care physician. He is on permanent disability but manages to live a more-than-humble lifestyle. He has developed a trusting relationship with the psychiatrist and finally admits that he sells his pain medications in order to pay his rent and car loan. He takes just enough of the prescribed pain medications to test positive on monthly toxicology screens that the primary care physician has instituted.

Scenario 8 A health promotion nurse and family medicine physician are conducting a smoking cessation class. The attendees begin to talk about their increased irritability and that they find themselves becoming easily frustrated. A single mother reports that her major stressor is her children, especially her 9-year-old son. She notes that he is upsetting her frequently with his behavior and that she is having urges to either smoke or choke the child to death. The urges have become so strong that she has twice had dreams about following through, and on one occasion she put her hands on his neck but did not squeeze.

Scenario 9 A physician treats a man and his wife separately in a general medicine clinic. The man discloses that he is having an affair with a same-sex partner and asks to be tested for sexually transmitted diseases. He reports that he "dabbles" in drug use, specifically methamphetamine, which his male partner supplies. Because of the high rate of unprotected sex and HIV among men who have sex with men using methamphetamine, the physician suspects that the man is at risk for HIV, hepatitis B, syphilis, and other sexually transmitted diseases. The physician believes that the man's wife is also at risk, because the couple continues to be sexually active and has not used condoms in many years. At the wife's next appointment, she asks the physician why her husband suddenly has decided to undergo "a bunch of medical tests" and asks if she should be aware of anything regarding her husband.

Acknowledgments The following authors contributed to the scenarios in this chapter: Laura Weiss Roberts, M.D., M.A., Daryn Reicherter, M.D., Jodi K. Casados, M.D., Joseph B. Layde, M.D., J.D., Celeste Lopez, M.D., Peter Marcus, M.S., M.A., Lawrence M. McGlynn, M.D., Richard Shaw, M.D., Christopher Warner, M.D., LTC, Mark Wright, M.D.

References

1. Schloendorff v. Society of New York Hospital, 105 N.E. 92 (N.Y., 1914).
2. Application of President and Directors of Georgetown College, 331 F.2d 1000 (D.C. Cir. 1964).
3. Strunk v. Strunk, 445 S.W.2d 145 (Ct. of Appeals, Ky. 1969).
4. In re Quinlan, 70 N.J. 10, 355 A.2d 647; 1976.
5. Superintendent of Belchertown State School & another v. Joseph Saikewicz, 370 N.E.2d 417 (Mass.,1977).
6. Cruzan by Cruzan v. Director, Missouri Department of Health, 497 U.S. 261; 1990.
7. "Nancy Cruzan Dies, Outlived by a Debate Over the Right to Die," New York Times, December 27; 1990.

8. Omnibus Budget Reconciliation Act of 1990, Pub. L. 101–508, 104 Stat. 1388; 1990.
9. 45 CFR 84.55.
10. Robertson, JA:. Extreme prematurity and parental rights after Baby Doe. 34 Hastings Center Report; 2004. 4, pp. 32–9.
11. Griswold v. Connecticut, 381 U.S. 479; 1965.
12. Roe v. Wade, 410 U.S. 113; 1973.
13. ORS (Oregon Revised Statutes)127.800-995; 1997.
14. Lessard v. Schmidt, 349 F.Supp. 1078 (E.D. Wis.1972)
15. Addington v. Texas, 441 U.S. 418; 1979.
16. Vitaly Tarasoff et al. v. The Regents of the University of California, 529 P.2d 533 (Cal.1974).
17. Vitaly Tarasoff et al. v. The Regents of the University of California, 551 P.2d 334 (Cal.1976).
18. 42 CFR Part 2.
19. Pub. L. No. 104–191, 110 Stat. 1936; 1996.
20. http://www.hhs.gov/ocr/privacy/hipaa/administrative/index.html. Accessed 6 Dec 2013.

Recommended Reading

Menikoff J. Law and bioethics: An introduction. Washington, DC: Georgetown University Press; 2001.
Roberts LW, Hoop JG. Professionalism and ethics: Q & A self-study guide for mental health professionals. Arlington: American Psychiatric Publishing; 2008.

Chapter 3
Multicultural and Ethical Considerations in American Medicine

Shashank V. Joshi, Daryn Reicherter, Andres J. Pumariega, and Laura Weiss Roberts

The United States is undergoing unprecedented growth in its social and demographic diversity. This growth comes from the expansion of peoples of non-European origins, both underrepresented minority individuals who were born in the United States and individuals who have migrated to the United States [1–3]. At the rate it is changing, the country will be a transgenerationally racial/ethnic/cultural plurality by the year 2042 – and for persons under the age of 18, by 2019. Many countries throughout the world are experiencing this "shifting demographic" phenomenon, which has awakened practitioners, teachers, and leaders throughout healthcare and medical education to the importance of knowledge, attitudes, and skills related to multiculturalism. To fulfill societal expectations of the medical profession will increasingly require attunement to patients: an appreciation for how culture shapes perspectives that influence the illness experience, the doctor-patient relationship, and engagement with the healthcare system.

S.V. Joshi, M.D. • D. Reicherter, M.D. • L.W. Roberts, M.D., M.A. (✉)
Department of Psychiatry and Behavioral Sciences,
Stanford University School of Medicine, Stanford, CA, USA
e-mail: RobertsL@stanford.edu

A.J. Pumariega, M.D.
Department of Psychiatry, Cooper Health System and Cooper
Medical School of Rowan University, Camden, NJ, USA

© Springer Science+Business Media New York 2015
L.W. Roberts, D. Reicherter (eds.), *Professionalism and Ethics in Medicine*,
DOI 10.1007/978-1-4939-1686-3_3

Multiculturalism in Clinical Care

Multiculturalism is based on the assumption that there is no single way to conceptualize human behavior or to explain the realities and experiences of diverse
cultural groups [2, 4]. In this framework, clinicians are asked to reflect on the observation that each individual has a unique story and that cultural meaning is woven
into that story, and each person, like a tapestry [5]. Indeed, in every encounter with
a patient, there are at least three separate cultures present and interacting: that of the
patient and family, that of the provider, and that of the medical or institutional culture where clinical work occurs. In this tripartite model, proposed by Tseng and
Streltzer [3], it becomes clear that every patient encounter involves mediating effectively ("cultural effectiveness") in relation to each cultural contribution that shapes
the interaction.

One culture participating in the interaction is that of the patient. Patients come to
the encounter with culturally shaped biases, assumptions, and beliefs that are not
always known to the provider but can influence the expectations and desired outcomes of the patient. The ethical principle of *Respect for Persons* is fulfilled when
providers can effectively work with patients and families with cultural backgrounds
different from that of the provider [6]. The patient's expectations of the physician,
motivation for treatment, explanation for the emergence of symptoms, and adherence with treatment recommendations can each be influenced by the patient's cultural background.

The second culture to consider in this exchange is the culture of the healthcare
provider. The sociodemographic background, life experience, personal beliefs, and
professional training of the provider will shape his or her interaction and communication with patients. Most medical providers are of Caucasian background, and
some groups (African-Americans, Latinos, and Native/Indigenous peoples) are
especially underrepresented in American medicine [7]. Even when many aspects of
the cultural background of the patient are similar to those of the clinician, differences are inevitable – and should be welcome.

The culture of American medicine, and its expression in the clinical care institution, is a third factor in each doctor-patient interaction. Most physicians and other
providers within an institution may become accustomed to both visible and invisi-
ble elements of the cultural environment of their workplace and may be unaware of
its collective influence on their practice [8]. Medical specialties, furthermore, each
have their own subcultures that include traditions, regulations, and attitudes, which
are not necessitated by specific medical knowledge: for example, whether physician, nurse, and care manager work together as equal team members or in more
hierarchical fashion depends on the past professional and training experiences of
each member, as well as the cultural milieu and other influences in the clinical and
societal setting. How patients and allied health personnel regard physicians may
vary by the dominant culture in that environment.

Given that many thousands of healthcare interactions occur each day and that
each is affected by the culture of the patient, the physician, and the immediate

context, the effectiveness of clinical care – as well as the ethics of clinical care – will be influenced by attentiveness to multiculturalism. Failure to appreciate the impact of culture may render useless or inaccessible what would otherwise be excellent care resources. Many barriers to care exist. Language differences serve as one example, but other less obvious barriers also arise – barriers related to lack of transportation, limited resources, inability to access and navigate health systems, and limited feelings of trust in healthcare institutions in the United States on the basis of previous experiences.

Other barriers to effective healthcare relate to beliefs about illness that are not aligned between the culture of Western medicine and the culture of the individual in need of care. For example, the notion of "germs" as a cause of disease is not universally held. The presumption that patients will agree with this "Western" explanation – and will therefore follow an evidence-based treatment plan – can lead to poor adherence and poor outcomes. These concerns may be greatest when the condition is very severe and highly stigmatized, such as with HIV infection or serious mental illness. In another example, many patients may receive treatment from non-Western practitioners. Some individuals may seek care in a Western medicine clinic and use acupuncture and herbal treatments in addition to or instead of prescribed pharmaceutical agents. Some people may receive treatment from a *curandero* (traditional healer in Latin American Culture), and others may see a *Kru Khmer* (traditional healer in Cambodian culture) rather than a Western practitioner. Moreover, some people may approach a Catholic priest and others may approach a Buddhist monk for a problem that they consider spiritual – a problem that a Western healthcare provider might see as a physical or mental health problem.

Beyond psychosocial issues related to culture in clinical care, biological considerations related to culture also factor into the provision of effective care for diverse patient populations. Healthcare providers must understand vulnerabilities with respect to specific illnesses and ethnicity. This concept is less about "cultural sensitivity" and more about understanding differential risk factors for disease, so as to appropriately care for high-risk individuals. For instance, some ethnic groups have a higher likelihood of developing diabetes and must, therefore, have their healthcare managed with special attention. Specific vulnerabilities and resilience patterns should be well understood by practitioners working with populations with differential susceptibility for disease. Some culturally supported behaviors around personal health, such as diet, physical activity, sexual behaviors, or alcohol consumption can influence risk level for specific healthcare issues. Immigration status and situation are also important. For instance, "refugee" status generally implies vulnerability to illness simply by the nature of events involved in refugee situations. Refugees may be more likely to experience physical injury, trauma, and sexual assault and, therefore, be at higher risk for the medical and psychiatric pathology associated with these experiences.

In sum, multiculturalism is a fact of present-day clinical medicine. Culturally informed care is more likely to be effective, and as discussed below, it is more likely to be ethically sound care. A cautionary note is necessary, however. While it is important to know about culture and culturally related risk factors, the encounter between physician and patient should be focused on the individual patient – not generalities, prejudices, and assumptions. For instance, consider the patient who is a "refugee from Iran." Incorrect assumptions may leap to the practitioner's mind: The patient is Farsi speaking. The patient is a Muslim. The patient has negative attitudes about Western culture. Assumptions like these are unhelpful at best and may be grossly inaccurate. The patient could very well be a non-Farsi-speaking non-Muslim with no specific preconceived notions about Western culture. Knowledge about political conditions in Iran and typical circumstances involved with refugee status from Iran may be helpful in establishing a therapeutic dialogue between provider and patient. But listening carefully and understanding the life circumstances *of the individual patient* are essential for the clinician – as a matter of professionalism – to be exceptionally attentive to the problems of conscious and unconscious bias in the care of this person. Approaching the individual patient in this manner is the basis of culturally informed care. This "patient-centered" approach also accommodates patients and families from cultural backgrounds where a more "doctor-centered" approach is preferred, in which the physician is more directive and the patient/family adopts a more passive role. Ultimately, a physician with high levels of adaptability will allow for rapid identification of patient/family preferences for shared decision-making and will readily incorporate these preferences into the care approach, even if the physician prefers an alternate model [9].

Models of Culturally Informed Care

Multiple models have been proposed to guide health professionals regarding culturally informed care. Two such models are the cultural competence model and the explanatory models approach. Both of these have merit and seek to elevate the role of culture in communication with patients and the development of treatment approaches that are respectful and helpful and avoid harm in the care of patients.

Cultural Competence Model

Terry Cross and his colleagues introduced the term *cultural competence* in their efforts to address the cultural needs of a growing population of diverse children and youth with serious emotional disturbance [10]. They defined *cultural competence* as the state of being capable to serve people from diverse cultural and socioeconomic backgrounds. They outlined components of knowledge, skill, attitudes, and values that both clinicians and the healthcare organizations they operate within should incorporate in order to operate effectively in a context of cultural difference. They outlined a cultural competence continuum where cultural competence is the last step toward an ideal state. This continuum is illustrated on a scale from cultural destructiveness to cultural proficiency, as shown in Figure 3.1, and can be translated into well-accepted bioethical values.

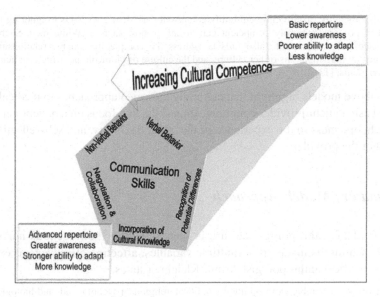

Fig. 3.1 Culturally competent communication: a skills-oriented developmental model (Reprinted with permission from [9].)

Although acknowledging that the concept of cultural competence may appeal to educators, some scholars point out that this term denotes a sort of "endpoint" and that this "mastery of a body of knowledge and skills … may insidiously lead us down the wrong path when applied to cross-cultural interactions. Culture is not a finite data set to be mastered, but instead a concept that is complex, dynamic, and individual" [11]. Further,

> Although our shared "medical culture" is based largely on achieving competence, we should take care when applying this term broadly to *mastering* other cultures [emphasis added]. We may find that competency-based education can be applied more easily to the domains of knowledge and skills than to attitudes. Communication skills built upon the attitudes of openness, flexibility, self-reflection, and, yes, *humility* are ultimately what will make individuals responsive and sensitive to the delivery of care to diverse populations. This is the framework medical educators should be striving to introduce, model reinforce, and evaluate. This is the path of lifelong learning about oneself in relation to others that is most fruitful. [11]

The term *cultural humility* [11, 12] is consistent with the concepts of self-reflection and self-critique, instead of mastery of sets of information. The physician who can be responsive and attuned to cultural nuances and differences is most likely to be able to incorporate information provided by patients and is less likely to leave sociocultural misunderstandings unaddressed. In this way, the physician can adduce an understanding of the patient's/family's situation from *their* point of view. Other authors caution against defining *culture* too narrowly [12].

> The somewhat abstract nature of the term *culture* often results in a workplace definition of culture that is narrow and concrete and reduces culture to ethnic minorities [only]. This type of thinking often leads to exempting providers from ethnic minority backgrounds from

the responsibility of providing culturally competent care. It further leads to ignoring the need to provide culturally competent care to all groups, such as White men. Such a restricted notion of culture also fails to address the complexities in the relationships between an individual, his or her culture, and the culture of biomedicine, which is alien to most patients. [13]

The above models highlight that culturally informed approaches to medical care feature basic patient/provider communication skills that focus on a patient-centered approach, openness to the experience of the other, flexibility, and self-reflection on the part of the provider.

Explanatory Models Approach

In the field of anthropology, culture is seen as neither homogenous nor static [12, 13]. Culture is made up of multiple variables, affecting all aspects of experience. As medical anthropologist Arthur Kleinman states:

> [Culture] is inseparable from economic, political, religious, psychological, and biological conditions. Culture is a process through which ordinary activities and conditions take on an emotional tone and a moral meaning for participants. ...Cultural processes frequently differ within the same ethnic or social group because of differences in age cohort, gender, political association, class, religion, ethnicity, and even personality. [14]

The shortcoming is that the medical field often falls into a categorical trap and may *equate* culture with ethnicity, nationality, and/or language. An example would be to assume that patients of a certain ethnicity are assumed to have a core set of beliefs about illness owing to ethnic traits.

> Cultural competency [then] becomes a series of "do's and don'ts" that define how to treat a patient of a given ethnic background... The idea of isolated societies with shared cultural meanings would be rejected by anthropologists, today, since it leads to dangerous stereotyping—such as, "Chinese believe this, "Japanese believe that," and so on—as if entire societies or ethnic groups could be described by these simple slogans. [14]

Kleinman introduced the explanatory models approach as an interview technique that seeks to clarify how the social world affects and is affected by illness within the context of an individual's life. His hope was that this approach would open clinicians to human communication and set their expert knowledge *alongside* the patient's own explanation and viewpoint (see Box 3.1).

> The explanatory models approach does not ask, for example, "What do Mexicans call this problem?" It asks, "What do you call this problem?" and thus a direct and immediate appeal is made to the patient as an individual, not as a representative of a group. ...one activity that even the busiest clinician should be able to find time to do ... [is] routinely ask patients (and where appropriate family members) what matters most to them in the experience of illness and treatment. The clinicians can then use that crucial information in thinking through treatment decisions and negotiating with patients. [14]

The *Diagnostic and Statistical Manual of Mental Disorders* (DSM), 5th edition [15], features a cultural formulation interview that can be adapted for different clinical

Box 3.1 The Explanatory Models Approach [14]

What do you call this problem?
What do you believe is the cause of this problem?
What course do you expect it to take? How serious is it?
What do you think this problem does inside your body? How does it affect
  your body and your mind?
What do you most fear about this condition?
What do you most fear about the treatment?

situations, including nonpsychiatric settings. Kleinman's explanatory models approach [14] expands upon the DSM cultural formulation and allows clinicians to create a short ethnography-like formulation.

Ethnography is a term from the field of anthropology that refers to the description of what life is like in the "local world" of the person (or patient) – usually one different from that of the anthropologist (or physician). It facilitates empathy with the patient's/family's lived experience of the illness and can lead to a narrative that ideally *conveys the clinical story* from the patient/family's worldview. The six steps in this ethnographic approach include the following [14]:

1. Asking about ethnic identity and whether it matters for the patient – for example, whether it is an important part of the patient's sense of self.
2. Evaluating what is at stake for the patient/family and their loved ones, which can include inquiring about close relationships, financial/material resources, and religious/spiritual beliefs and shed light on the moral lives of patients/families.
3. Constructing the "illness narrative" on the basis of a series of questions (Box 3.1) to understand the meaning of illness. Explanatory models can be used to open up a conversation on cultural meanings that have clinical relevance.
4. Considering the current stressors and social supports in patients'/families' lives.
5. Examining the influence of culture on the clinical relationship. An important ethnographic tool is self-reflection regarding the intersection of the world of the physician and the world of the patient. Kleinman reminds us, "Teaching practitioners to consider the effects of the culture of biomedicine is contrary to the view of the expert as authority and to the media's view that technical expertise is always the best answer" [13].
6. Considering how relevant cultural issues are to a particular clinical situation. This vital step asks whether too much attention to potential cultural differences with the provider could be experienced by the patients and families as intrusive and could even lead to a sense of being singled out and stigmatized or could lead to a misdiagnosis.

The culturally competent communication model proposed by Teal and Street [9] integrates existing frameworks for cultural competence and explanatory models including culture in patient care, with models of effective patient-centered communication. In this model there are four critical elements of culturally competent communication in the medical encounter: communication repertoire, situational awareness, adaptability, and acknowledging core cultural issues. The approach includes key communication skills such as the incorporation of cultural knowledge, recognition of potential differences, verbal and nonverbal behaviors, and negotiation and collaboration. These elements are seen as fundamental to acquisition of more skills corresponds to increasing complexity and culturally competent communication (Fig. 3.1).

The cultural competence model and the explanatory models approach provide pathways that allow for cultural engagement, with the intention of focusing on the individual and providing the most attuned and astute care to help address the needs he or she presents. *Respect for Persons* and *Beneficence* are thus the basis of culturally informed patient care. Kleinman offers the recommendation that the first ethical tasks for clinicians are to *acknowledge* and *understand* the moral meaning of suffering for any given patient.

> This is much different than cultural competency. Finding out what matters most to another person is not a technical skill. It is an elective affinity to the patient. …It is what Franz Kafka said a "born doctor" has: "a hunger for people" … And its main thrust is to focus on the patient as an individual, not a stereotype; as a human being facing danger and uncertainty, not merely a case; as an opportunity for the doctor to engage in an essential moral task, not an issue in cost-accounting. [14]

Practical Solutions for Clinical Effectiveness in Cross-Cultural Settings

In addition to adopting cultural formulation models, healthcare providers have practical methods for becoming effective in cross-cultural situations. Cultural competence training can be helpful, if conducted skillfully. There are continuing medical education (CME) credits in cultural sensitivity or cultural effectiveness. Such education units may be general to learning about how to become more effective or specific to learning more about a particular culture and its relation to medical practice. CME units on cultural sensitivity are becoming more common with the changing demographic in the United States.

Specific cultural understanding can also be very helpful. Much insight may be gained in learning about the culture and history of a specific group. Furthermore, insights into that culture's model for disease and its perception of effective treatment may help healthcare providers to be more effective in understanding the perspective of their patients and discussing treatment plans. Also, consultation on cultural issues is appropriate – it may be considered similar to consulting with a healthcare colleague with a different specialty. When possible, it is very appropriate

Box 3.2 The LEARN Model of Cross-Cultural Communication [22]

Listen with sympathy and empathy to the patient's perception of the problem
Explain your perception of the problem
Acknowledge and discuss differences and similarities
Recommend treatment
Negotiate agreement

and perhaps essential to have a discussion with a cultural broker; to gain insight into a case in which a cultural issue has the practitioner frustrated is very appropriate and possibly essential. If a healthcare provider is working with many patients with a similar, collective psycho-social experience, the provider can improve effectiveness by learning more about the realities and/or risks associated with that particular experience. For example, healthcare providers working with refugee patients would benefit greatly by learning about the experience of refugees, the common psychosocial circumstances refugees face, and the increased risks for illness they have because of their experience.

Working effectively in cross-cultural settings often includes working through translated language. Language translation should be provided by a professional interpreter whenever possible. It is not uncommon to have language translated through family members or friends, but this is not ideal for many reasons. Professional interpreters are trained to convey exactly what a healthcare provider says into the patient's language and what the patient says into the healthcare provider's language. They do not take liberties with concepts being translated, except when specifically indicated. They provide literal translation between languages. Some healthcare settings are fortunate enough to have staff with capabilities in the language of the cultures served. This is ideal because often the bilingual provider understands both perspectives as well as both languages. They can translate concepts. They can also provide cultural consultation and help bring provider and patient to common understanding. In such instances, it is important to make sure that the interpreters are well trained in relevant clinical issues. Their understanding is important for ideal communication.

In working with culturally diverse populations, it is absolutely essential to create very clear treatment plans based on accurate communication (Boxes 3.2 and 3.3). Ensuring that the patient understands the assessment and treatment plan may require some extra work in a translated, intercultural case – but this is necessary for effectiveness and must include the patient's understanding of the diagnosis and plan for intervention. Assumptions from the patient or the provider can lead to miscommunication and poor follow-through. Coordinating treatment plans with other providers in such cases may prove to be effective.

Box 3.3 The RESPECT Model of Cross-Cultural Communication [23]

- *Rapport*

  - Connect on a social level
  - Seek the patient's point of view
  - Consciously attempt to suspend judgment
  - Recognize and avoid making assumptions

- *Empathy*

  - Remember that the patient has come to you for help
  - Seek out and understand the patient's rationale for his or her behaviors or illness
  - Verbally acknowledge and legitimize the patient's feelings

- *Support*

  - Ask about and try to understand barriers to care and compliance
  - Help the patient overcome barriers
  - Involve family members if appropriate
  - Reassure the patient you are and will be available to help

- *Partnership*

  - Be flexible with regard to issues of control
  - Negotiate roles when necessary
  - Stress that you will be working together to address medical problems

- *Explanations*

  - Check often for understanding
  - Use verbal clarification techniques

- *Cultural competence*

  - Respect the patient and his or her culture and beliefs
  - Understand that the patient's view of you may be identified by ethnic or cultural stereotypes
  - Be aware of your own biases and preconceptions
  - Know your limitations in addressing medical issues across cultures
  - Understand your personal style and recognize when it may not be working with a given patient

- *Trust*

  - Self-disclosure may be an issue for some patients who are not accustomed to Western medical approaches
  - Take the necessary time and consciously work to establish trust

Examples of Ethical Issues in Culturally Informed Patient Care

Ethical practice guides health professionals to respect and honor a patient's cultural beliefs and practices, even when there are differences, barriers, and challenges. This aspiration is admirable, but there are many situations in which the cultural dimensions of a patient's care may introduce unexpected ethical tensions that are difficult to resolve. Among the examples described and illustrated below are cultural considerations and acceptance of treatment; values differences related to individualism, autonomy, and collectivism; linguistic support and confidentiality; modesty versus the need for thoroughness; and behavior that does not conform to Western normative expectations.

Cultural Considerations and Treatment Acceptability

On one hand, conflict may occur between the medical team and the patient if his or her culturally sanctioned treatment preferences are at odds with standard practice in Western medicine. On the other hand, a patient may refuse standard treatments practiced by Western medicine due to the perception that such treatments may violate their cultural beliefs and values or put them in loyalty conflicts with cultural healers or traditional family members [6].

> **Illustration 1. Constructive compromise.**
> The parents of a 16-year-old immigrant female from Mexico took her to see a pediatrician for worsening symptoms of depression. The parents did not mention that they had taken her to a *curandero* (cultural healer) who had recommended pursuing a ritual for addressing possession by an evil spirit. The pediatrician recommended combined psychotherapy and pharmacotherapy for her treatment. The young woman was very much in favor of the pediatrician's recommendation. She attended a few visits with a psychiatrist and began to show improvement. Pressure from her father led her to drop out of treatment out of a concern that the cultural healer would see him as not in charge of his family. The pediatrician followed up with the family and encouraged the young woman to return into treatment, with the compromise that she see the psychiatrist only for pharmacotherapy while the healer saw her for spiritual counseling.

The compromise in the case illustrates the utility of not only recommending treatment but also negotiating a treatment pathway that has a high degree of likely adherence, on the basis of the preferences and customs of the patient and family.

Individualism and Autonomy Versus Collective Identity

Because Western culture tends to value individualism over collectivism, problems can arise when the medical team wishes to honor the ethical principle of autonomy if the patient is from a culture that views the family as the essential unit of society [6]. For example, the family of an adult patient who is capable of informed consent may feel they have the right to view the confidential treatment record or to make decisions for the patient with regard to disclosing the diagnosis. The issue may get even more complicated with adolescent patients, where the principles of *autonomy, beneficence,* and *confidentiality* may all be tested. Because of the tensions of consent, disclosure, and the role of the family, the American Academy of Child and Adolescent Psychiatry has developed a Code of Ethics that states, in summary, "The wellbeing, functioning, and development of youth as individuals, and as a group, should be optimized whenever appropriate. Societal, familial, and other group pressures should not override the best interest of the child" [16].

Illustration 2. Nonadherence to treatment.
A 7-year-old boy was seen by his pediatrician for an evaluation for disruptive behavioral problems, and he was at risk for expulsion from school. The pediatrician obtained rating scales from teachers and the mother and reviewed a school counselor's report, all of which were consistent with a diagnosis of attention-deficit disorder. The boy was clearly hyperactive and inattentive in the office environment, though quite pleasant in his demeanor. The pediatrician recommended a trial of a stimulant medication, reviewed risks and benefits, obtained signed consent, and gave the mother a prescription as well as symptom rating scales to evaluate baseline and treatment response. The pediatrician did not inquire about cultural considerations in accepting treatment. The mother, a 24-year-old Afghan woman, lived with her extended family. The grandmother protested that the doctor was going to turn the child into an "addict" and summarily flushed the medications down the commode.

Linguistic Support Versus Confidentiality

Patients with limited English proficiency often need interpretation for effective patient education and engagement and to obtain appropriate informed consent. Many healthcare organizations, in spite of government requirements, often do not have sufficient professional linguistic support resources (i.e., professional interpreters trained in the language and medical content matter and bound by confidentiality oaths). It is not unusual for many patients and clinicians to request and rely on friends or relations of the patient for interpretation or for clinicians to engage hospital personnel in this task who may be from the patient's community.

Illustration 3. Confidentiality in the context of stigma.
Trahn is a 32-year-old Vietnamese immigrant male with limited English proficiency who finally visited a primary care physician at the urging of his secret male partner due to his concerns about having contracted HIV during a one-night encounter with another man. Trahn had never "come out" to his family, even though he lived with them, expecting rejection if they knew of his sexual orientation and behavior. He did not go to the Vietnamese community clinic in his neighborhood for fear that his family might find out about his "secrets." The primary care physician spoke no Vietnamese and proceeded to let him know that he was calling for an interpreter from the community. While Trahn waited, he was quite anxious but could not communicate his fear that this interpreter might know him or his family.

A simple inquiry into the acceptability (or not) of this plan – for instance, "How does this plan sound to you?" – may have avoided the anxiety-provoking situation for the patient. Such an inquiry can also convey cultural attunement that can enhance the provider-patient treatment alliance (and subsequent treatment adherence).

Modesty Versus Thorough Examination, Diagnosis, and Intervention

Some cultures prescribe strict gender separation, especially with women in regard to physical examination, with only female clinicians being allowed to provide these services.

Illustration 4. Cultural barriers in an emergency.
A Saudi woman and her husband came into the emergency department after a serious motor vehicle crash. The husband was slightly injured, but his wife had severe internal injuries, and her blood pressure was dropping rapidly. Though there were female nurses present, the husband strongly objected to the trauma team cutting off the woman's clothes to examine her. He refused to consider life-saving interventions. When the couple's daughter arrived, he was calmer and cooperative.

In this scenario, it would have been useful for one member of the team to guide the husband through what would occur and accommodate certain modesty practices where possible, such as minimizing exposure of her body to male staff members, and explain the seriousness/life-threatening nature of the situation.

Culturally Normative Behaviors Conflicting with Western Societal Norms

Ethical issues may arise when Western practitioners observe evidence of exposure to culturally sanctioned practices that are not in keeping with Western medical practice. The perception that a culturally normal behavior is irrational or even harmful may necessitate that a clinician make a determination of whether the offending issue is evidence of abuse at a level that must be reported.

Illustration 5. Complementary treatment.
A 35-year-old Khmer woman presents to the urgent care clinic with a very high fever. She appears very anxious. She says that she had sought care from a Kru Khmer (traditional healer) earlier that day but feared that the treatment had not worked. The doctor performs a physical examine on her. She has deep, red marks on her forehead and forearms and large circular bruises on her back. She says that they are from "cupping" and explains that the healers commonly will use coining or cupping for fever.

In areas with large Southeast Asian populations, physicians may see signs of coining and cupping regularly. These are common, culturally-sanctioned folk treatments for somatic symptoms in people from Southeast Asia. The physical marks on a patient's body can be alarming. Even when the practice is explained, Western healthcare professionals may not understand what they see from the patient's point of view. If a physician sees these marks, he or she must make sure that no abuse is present, i.e., that the adult patient had sought the alternative treatment voluntarily.

Effective Approaches to Address Ethical Situations in a Multicultural Environment

The concept of ethically astute and culturally informed care refers to the ability to engage effectively with, and provide quality healthcare to, an ever-more diverse range of patients and families. Culturally attuned communication, improved patient satisfaction, treatment adherence, and clinical outcomes are linked and supported by vigorous efforts in cross-cultural education. Two influential Institute of Medicine Reports, *Unequal Treatment* [17], published in 2002, and *Crossing the Quality Chasm* [18], published in 2001, have emphasized that patient and family-centered care and cultural competence are crucial to achieve equity, improve quality, and reduce significant racial and ethnic disparities in healthcare today. Clinically astute care is thus predicated on the ethical principles of *Respect for Persons, Beneficence,* and *Justice.*

Some governmental and professional bodies have also begun to codify best practices, standards, and guidelines for culturally informed care, to guide clinicians in addressing the cultural needs of their diverse patients. These "best practice" documents have included the Cultural Competence Standards for Managed Care Mental Health for Four Racial/Ethnic Underserved/Underrepresented Populations [19] and the National Culturally and Linguistically Appropriate Services (CLAS) Standards in Health and Health Care [20]. The American Academy of Child and Adolescent Psychiatry has also developed the Practice Parameter for Cultural Competence in Child and Adolescent Psychiatric Practice [21], which outlines recommendations for culturally informed care that are easily adaptable to the rest of medicine. These guidelines are oriented to reduce health disparities for diverse populations, to improve the working alliance, and to maximize the effectiveness of treatment.

Culturally attuned clinicians may be able to anticipate ethical issues and clarify in advance how the patient would like these issues to be handled [6]. Providers who are well versed in ethical guidelines across the lifespan will be much better equipped to anticipate such pitfalls and proactively inquire about individual and cultural norms in a particular clinical situation. Beyond knowledge of guidelines, ethical "best practices" include, for example, ongoing or continuing education to enhance understanding of specific cultures and to improve communication skills in a cross-cultural context. Other optimal approaches include use of well-prepared translators and engagement of cultural consultants or "wise people" who can help clarify the intent, hopes, and experiences of patients. The ultimate aim of culturally informed care is true attunement to the individual in need, fulfilling the fundamental ethical principles of medicine.

Review and Reflect: Ask Yourself and Talk with Colleagues

For each of the following scenarios, ask yourself and talk with colleagues about the following questions: What ethical tensions exist in this situation? What legal obligations, if any, are present? What are the culturally important dimensions depicted in the scenario? What are the clinician's next steps?

Scenario 1 During a 1-month postoperative checkup following a total colectomy, a patient who is a Bosnian refugee wants to give his surgeon a gift as a token of his appreciation, a $20 bottle of brandy. His quality of life has improved substantially after many years of severe abdominal pain from ulcerative colitis. A Bosnian translator/cultural broker explains to the surgeon that he would offend the patient if he rejected the gift. The surgeon is often offered gifts from patients, but is particularly concerned in this case because he knows that a $20 gift for this patient is a considerable sacrifice.

Scenario 2 A middle-aged Hispanic veteran who has seen an internist at the VA primary care clinic for over a year has many gastrointestinal complaints, which have been thoroughly worked up. The results of these investigations have essentially been normal, and no obvious physical abnormality is contributing to his symptoms. During his last visit, the veteran also reported difficulty sleeping and drinking more alcohol lately. He demanded a CT of his stomach, and when the internist recommended he see the clinic psychologist to rule out depression, the man became very upset and filed a complaint with the patient advocate.

Scenario 3 A married couple present for medical care at a clinic where patients and staff represent many different demographics. They meet with the clinic's social worker for their intake. The wife requests a female primary care physician and is assigned to one of the clinic's female physicians. The husband is not particular about the gender of the physician, but because of reasons he refuses to disclose, he states, "I don't want a gay doctor." The social worker asks the clinic director for advice.

Scenario 4 A Burmese refugee with a history of severe migraine headaches is highly symptomatic with a low level of functioning, but does not adhere to either preventive or acute treatment recommendations from his neurologist. He also has a poor attendance record for his English language class. He asks the neurologist to fill out immigration paperwork that would waive his ability to take his citizenship exam on the basis that he cannot learn English because the severe migraines prevent him from being able to concentrate for long periods of time. The neurologist wonders how to respond.

Scenario 5 A patient comes into his clinic appointment very upset, stating that he was approached in the waiting room by someone who appeared to be another doctor and said, "Jesus supports you, and will help you."

Scenario 6 A physician is approached by one of his chronically ill immigrant patients for some "lunch money." The physician is aware of the financial difficulties of the patient, but does not want to set an uncomfortable precedent in their relationship – particularly because he sees the patient often, not only in the clinic but in the local neighborhood.

Scenario 7 A patient asks her physician for a "work excuse" so that she may attend a political rally in the state capital. The rally relates to a recent controversy in the state budget and union collective bargaining rights. She is a teacher and states the uncertainty surrounding her job has made her extremely anxious. She makes the connection between the "work excuse" and her overall well-being and believes that the physician "must help" her. She states adamantly, "It's not just my job - my health is at stake!" The patient is first-generation Hispanic, originally from Mexico, and English is a second language for her. The physician is also Hispanic, but third generation and of South American origin.

Scenario 8 A psychiatrist evaluates a homeless, English-speaking man identifying as Native American. The patient describes having special relationships with crows. He believes that he can communicate with them through telepathy. He receives "special messages" from birds that influence his behavior. He reports further bizarre delusions around his magical influences over nature. His hygiene is poor, and he is malodorous. He has very odd habits around eating because of auditory hallucinations, and he is not getting enough nutrition and losing weight. He looks emaciated. He does not have a reasonable plan for shelter and sleeps "in a field." The psychiatrist hospitalizes the man with an involuntary hold for "grave disability" with the diagnosis of a psychotic disorder. Quickly, the hospital releases him. The discharge summary indicates the opinion that the patient's behaviors are "culturally appropriate." The patient returns to homelessness, untreated.

Scenario 9 A family physician works at a community health center that treats primarily Southeast Asian refugee and immigrant populations. A very experienced Cambodian language interpreter informs the physician that he is a leader in the Cambodian community and that he feels it is important to translate not only what the patients are saying but also what he knows about their current social situations.

Acknowledgments The following authors contributed to the scenarios in this chapter: Laura Weiss Roberts, M.D., M.A., Daryn Reicherter, M.D., Richard Balon, M.D., Shaili Jain, M.D., Steven B. McCann, M.D., Lawrence M. McGlynn, M.D.

References

1. Pumariega A, Joshi SV. Culture and development in children and youth. Child Adolesc Psychiatric Clin N Am. 2010;19:661–80.
2. McLoyd VC. Socioeconomic disadvantage and child development. Am Psychol. 1998;53(2):185–204.
3. Tseng WS, Streltzer J, editors. Cultural competence in clinical psychiatry. Washington, DC: American Psychiatric Publishing; 2004. p. 2–6.
4. Sholevar GP. Cultural child and adolescent psychiatry. In: Martin A, Volkmar F, editors. Lewis's child and adolescent psychiatry: a comprehensive textbook. Philadelphia: Lippincott, Williams and Wilkins; 2007. p. 57–65.
5. United States Census Bureau: American Community Survey. http://www.census.gov/acs/www/index.html. Accessed 12 May 2014.
6. Comas-Diaz L. Cross-cultural mental health treatment. In: Comas-Diaz L, Griffith E, editors. Clinical guidelines in cross-cultural mental health. New York: Wiley; 1988. p. 335–61.
7. Association of American Medical Colleges: Diversity in Medical Education: Facts & Figures 2012. https://members.aamc.org/eweb/DynamicPage.aspx?Action=Add&ObjectKeyF rom=1A83491A-9853-4C87-86A4-F7D95601C2E2&WebCode=PubDetailAdd&DoNotSave =yes&ParentObject=CentralizedOrderEntry&ParentDataObject=Invoice%20Detail&ivd_ formkey=69202792-63d7-4ba2-bf4e-a0da41270555&ivd_prc_prd_key=E1A7507B-F47B-40D0-8946-9ADBAB417F3E. Accessed 15 May 2014.
8. Betancourt J, Cervantes MC. Cross-cultural medical education in the US: key principles and experiences. Kaohsiung J Med Sci. 2009;25(9):471–8.
9. Teal CR, Street RL. Critical elements of culturally competent communication in the medical encounter: a review and model. Soc Sci Med. 2009;68(3):533–43.
10. Cross TL, Bazron BJ, Dennis KW, Isaacs MR. Toward a culturally competent system of care: a monograph on effective services for minority children who are severely emotionally disturbed. Washington, DC: CASSP Technical Assistance Center, Georgetown University Child Development Center; 1989.

11. Hixon A. Beyond cultural competence. Acad Med. 2003;78(6):634.
12. Dogra N, Karnik N. The cultural sensibility model: a process-oriented approach for children and adolescents. Child Adolesc Psychiatric Clin N Am. 2010;19:719–37.
13. Engebretson J, Mahoney J, Carlson ED. Cultural competence in the era of evidence-based practice. J Prof Nurs. 2008;24(3):172–8.
14. Kleinman A, Benson P. Anthropology in the clinic: the problem of cultural competency and how to fix it. PLoS Med. 2006;3(10):1673–6.
15. American Psychiatric Association. Diagnostic and statistical manual of mental disorders. 5th ed. Washington, DC: American Psychiatric Association; 2013.
16. Goldsmith M, Joshi SV. Ethical considerations in child and adolescent psychiatry. FOCUS. 2012;X(3):315–20.
17. Institute of Medicine, Committee on Understanding and Eliminating Racial and Ethnic Disparities in Health Care, Smedley BD, Stith AY, Nelson AR, editors. Unequal treatment: confronting racial and ethnic disparities in health care. Washington, DC: National Academy Press; 2002.
18. Institute of Medicine, Committee on Quality of Health Care in America. Crossing the quality chasm: a new health system for the 21st century. Washington, DC: National Academy Press; 2001.
19. U.S. Department of Health and Human Services. Four racial/ethnic panels: cultural competence standards for managed care mental health for four racial/ethnic underserved/underrepresented populations. Rockville: Center for Mental Health Services, Substance Abuse and Mental Health Administration; 2000.
20. U.S. Department of Health and Human Services. Office of minority health: national culturally and linguistically appropriate services (CLAS) standards in health and health care. Rockville: Office of Minority Health; 2000.
21. Pumariega AJ, Rothe E, Mian A, Carlisle L, Toppelberg C, Harris T, et al. Practice parameter for cultural competence in child and adolescent psychiatric practice. J Am Acad Child Adolesce Psychiatry. 2013;52(10):1101–15.
22. Berlin EA, Fowkes WC. A teaching framework for cross-cultural health care. Application in family practice. West J Med. 1983;139:934–8.
23. Welch M. Enhancing awareness and improving cultural competence in health care. A partnership guide for teaching diversity and cross-cultural concepts in heath professional training. San Francisco: University of California at San Francisco; 1998.

Recommended Reading

Fadiman A. The spirit catches you and you fall down: A Hmong child, her American doctors, and the collision of two cultures. New York: Farrar, Straus and Giroux; 1998.
Hoop JG, DiPasquale T, Hernandez J, Roberts LW. Ethics and culture in mental health care. Ethics Behav. 2008;18(4):353–72.
Kleinman A. The illness narratives: Suffering, healing, and the human condition. New York: Basic Books; 1989. Reprint edition.
Roberts LW, Battaglia J, Smithpeter M, Epstein RS. An office on main street: health care dilemmas in small communities. Hastings Cent Rep. 1999;29(4):28–37.

Chapter 4
Ethical Issues in Biomedical Research and Clinical Training

Laura Weiss Roberts, Maurice M. Ohayon, and Jane Paik Kim

Physicians and physicians-in-training encounter a variety of ethical issues in biomedical research and education conducted at their medical schools and affiliated hospitals. The ethical commitments of human research overlap to a great extent with the ethical commitments of clinical care, but there are some differences. For example, the clinical investigator must fulfill the standards of the profession as he or she seeks new knowledge of potential benefit to society and yet cannot guarantee benefit to each volunteer who enrolls in a clinical research protocol. A clinician, on the other hand, must fulfill the standards of the profession as he or she seeks to apply knowledge to benefit each patient. These two commitments are similar but not identical. In clinical training, many difficult ethical issues arise, primarily related to the role of the learner who has not yet mastered clinical medicine but can progressively and with supervision provide care with more and more independence and skill. The well-being of the patient remains foremost, but the aim of the physician-in-training to attain competence is another influence – and, according to some, a potential competing interest – in the academic medical training environment. In this chapter we outline many of the ethical issues in human research and clinical training that are relevant to physicians and physicians-in-training.

L.W. Roberts, M.D., M.A. (✉) • M.M. Ohayon, M.D., D.Sc., Ph.D. • J.P. Kim, Ph.D.
Department of Psychiatry and Behavioral Sciences,
Stanford University School of Medicine, Stanford, CA, USA
e-mail: RobertsL@stanford.edu

© Springer Science+Business Media New York 2015
L.W. Roberts, D. Reicherter (eds.), *Professionalism and Ethics in Medicine*,
DOI 10.1007/978-1-4939-1686-3_4

Biomedical Research Ethics

Principles

Respect for Persons, Beneficence, and *Justice* are the three principles that serve as the foundation for ethically sound human research. These principles were articulated in the Belmont Report of the National Commission for Protection of Human Subjects of Biomedical and Behavioral Research [1] nearly four decades ago and thereafter have had an enduring influence on all human subjects regulations in the United States. *Respect for Persons* is a principle that honors the dignity and underscores the autonomy of individuals who volunteer for human studies. *Beneficence* is the principle that affirms the health professional's duty to pursue "good," namely, knowledge that will be helpful to others in society. *Justice,* the third principle, signifies the commitment to the equitable distribution of burdens and benefits in society, that is, helping to ensure that the group or population bearing the greatest burden for research also derive benefit from it. All three principles, in concert, help to ensure that especially vulnerable individuals or groups are not taken advantage of, or exploited, in the research situation.

In recent years, two other ethics principles have been increasingly recognized for their centrality in ethically sound human studies. These two principles are *Veracity* and *Integrity* – notions that are perhaps presumed but are certainly in close alignment with the Belmont "triad." *Veracity* is the ethical commitment to be honest and not engage in deception. *Integrity* is the commitment to adhere wholly to the accepted standards of a profession, subordinating personal interests to the obligations of one's professional role. These two principles further buttress the ethical conduct of human studies and help to clarify why, for example, research that involves deception, such as occurred in the Tuskegee and Human Radiation, Humphreys', Milgram's, and Willowbrook experiments [2] – even if it generates new knowledge of value to society – is not ethically acceptable. Similarly, concerns about misconduct and conflicts of interest that may distort the judgment and practices of investigators have led to the heightened emphasis on research integrity [3]. Attitudes regarding the ethics of human research have advanced so much that present-day students may wonder why such concerns exist, but lessons of recent history suggest that ongoing attention to these issues is warranted.

Research safeguards and practices evolve as societal attitudes and values change and as science itself changes and creates new ethical questions. In the middle of the last century, for example, the societal focus on scientific discovery and the quest for new knowledge dominated views of human research. Investigators were held to the professional standards of rigor and truthfulness, certainly, but there was less emphasis – when compared to present day – on other issues, such as the safety of human subjects, the respect shown to volunteers in the research process, issues of fairness and discrimination, and conflicts of role and interest. Concerns about the exploitation of human beings in research are counterbalanced, however, by views regarding the importance of biomedical science in addressing human disease and suffering. With the crisis in the mid-1980s as HTLV-3, known today as HIV, was recognized, access to clinical research became recast for many as a societal "right." A similar set of attitudes now is evident in broad campaigns for research related to breast cancer, autism, and many other illnesses and conditions [4].

As science progresses, new ethical standards for science also advance. One illustration of this point relates to genetic investigation. Cloning and the use of human stem cells have received much attention, for instance, both in medicine and the popular media because these topics raise important questions about the nature of humanity and life itself. Less celebrated but still ethically challenging are issues related to confidentiality and the boundaries of informed consent when gathering genetic data in research – data that can reveal much about individuals and their families and create unanticipated psychosocial risks for them, now and in the future. Other ethical issues will arise with greater possibilities in the present era of personalized medicine and increased use of electronic medical record systems by clinicians and investigators to tailor treatment decisions. An example is the recent increasing presence of clinical trial designs taking an adaptive, "learn as we go" spirit. It is a commonly stated concern that ethics are "subjective" and "a moving target" – we suggest instead that ethical considerations in human studies are in fact rigorous; are based in fundamental, enduring principles; and operate in alignment with progress in society and science.

Safeguards and Practices

Ethical research embodies the Belmont principles of *Respect for Persons, Beneficence,* and *Justice,* as well as *Veracity* and *Integrity.* These ideals find their translation into real life through evolving and exacting safeguards, defined in federal human subjects regulations and enacted every day through professional practices.

In evaluating whether a particular research project is ethically sound, many features of the protocol should be taken into consideration. For instance, Table 4.1 shows how regulated safeguards and professional practices combine to protect human volunteers from unnecessary risk and ensure their respectful treatment in a clinical research protocol. It is important to note that the question under study and the context of the protocol are ethically important – not just the protocol itself. For example, the study should be grounded in a question that has significance. The investigative team should have adequate expertise, and the project should be designed in a manner that will produce information of some value, whether for people with a particular illness or for society at large. Stated differently, if a project does not have significance, it may not be appropriately executed, and if it is not well designed, why would it ever be ethically correct to ask a human subject to participate?

Table 4.1 Examples of safeguards across the course of protocol development, implementation, and follow-up

Assembly of scientific team to ensure appropriate content and methodological expertise
Training of scientific team and research staff regarding professionalism and ethics standards
Selection of scientific design and methodology to optimize meaningful findings and minimize risk
Scientific peer review, institutional review, and oversight
Conflict of interest management
Inclusion of least vulnerable population
Careful subject selection and recruitment procedures
Careful informed consent procedures
Inclusion of appropriate alternative decision-makers when needed
Appropriate environment/facilities for research to ensure physical and psychological safety of participants
Confidentiality protections for participants
Safety monitoring by research staff and oversight committees
Use of appropriate exit criteria to disenroll participants when necessary
Careful protection of data derived from the project
Rigorous scientific peer review of data-based manuscripts/presentations
Use of appropriate authorship standards

Similarly, it is important to consider whether the question could be addressed in a manner that is less risky for participants and whether every effort has been made to minimize the burdens and potential harms that participants may experience. Moreover, it must be asked if the protocol could pose greater risk than the underlying issue to be studied. When investigating whether an innovative treatment works for a disease, does every arm of the study meet "treatment as usual" or appropriate standards of care, and if not, what is the justification and what safeguards are in place? One should think carefully, for instance, about whether the protocol's informed consent procedure is sufficient, whether a mechanism for monitoring participant safety is in place (e.g., a Data Safety and Monitoring Board), and what "rescue" criteria and methods have been built into the protocol. Explicitly considering such questions is important for investigators and those entrusted with institutional oversight of human studies, but it is also essential for learners in medicine as one element of scientific literacy.

Many different safeguards exist and are vital to the current conduct of science involving human subjects. A human subject is defined in the federal regulations [5] as a living individual about whom an investigator conducting research obtains data through intervention or interaction with the individual or through identifiable private information. All research involving human subjects must be evaluated, or formally deemed exempt, by an Institutional Review Board (IRB). These institutional committees prospectively review protocols to ensure that a project has scientific merit, study participants are protected, and the investigative team has sufficient expertise to perform the work. IRBs intentionally have diverse representation from different scientific areas, and they also have community members bringing broader perspectives to the committee's decision-making process. IRBs are responsible for approving, or not approving, protocols – and they can intervene in ongoing protocols to modify or discontinue them. The level of oversight provided by an IRB is based, in general terms, on the level of risk and the balance of benefit and risk posed by the study, for example, "minimal risk," "increment above minimal risk," and "no prospect for direct benefit." With a minimal risk study and strong confidentiality safeguards built into a protocol, an IRB chair may make the decision of whether a protocol can be deemed exempt from IRB oversight or given approval to proceed, for example. Higher-risk studies involving special or protected groups will have full committee review and discussion before approval. Discontinuing an approved protocol is rare but may occur under many different circumstances. Early termination of a protocol can occur if the IRB or another specially designated oversight committee determines that the protocol is being conducted incorrectly or if the nature and/or number of adverse events is too great, new information arises that suggests the protocol places volunteers at risk for harm, or the team is not adhering to the proposed protocol.

Informed consent has a crucial role as a safeguard in human research as it does in clinical care. Ethically acceptable research is founded on the idea that a well-informed and decisionally capable person may choose to be in research and make this decision in a manner that is deliberate and in partnership with scientists who are seeking an answer to a question of importance to the volunteer and to society. Informed consent, to fulfill this idea, should not be seen as a single, "legalistic," or even transactional event – like signing a contract to buy a car or a condominium – but, rather, a dialogue-based process that is highly and sufficiently informative and allows the individual to make the decision authentically and in the absence of coercion. Informed consent thus stands on the pillars of appropriate information sharing, decisional capacity, and voluntariness. Decisional capacity is, in turn, based on four subcomponents or capacities: to communicate, to understand, to reason, and to appreciate in relation to the decision at hand. The level of decisional capacity is contingent upon the nature of the decision and the risks and benefits to be undertaken. In other words, for minimal risk research with some likelihood of benefit, an individual with reduced decisional abilities may be fully capable of consent. A more rigorous standard is applied for higher-risk research with little prospect for direct benefit.

Challenges in informed consent in human research have been carefully documented [6–9]. It is important to ensure that the potential participant understand the difference between research and usual clinical care and, as a corollary, the difference in the role of the clinical investigator and the usual "doctor." The therapeutic misconception [6], as some believe, is the idea held by research volunteers that the protocol "guarantees" essentially state-of-the-art care and likely benefit for the participant – no matter what the consent form says. A second challenge in informed consent is determining how much information is enough information. Most IRBs have taken the path of requiring lengthy consent forms to ensure that every possible outcome and adverse effect is anticipated and reviewed with the prospective volunteer. A third challenge is evaluating whether the prospective participant is capable of providing a decision that is truly voluntary. As one of us (LWR) wrote elsewhere:

> Voluntarism is a difficult concept to operationalize, because there are so many subtle influences upon an individual's true ability to make fully independent decisions and to act freely in certain situations or at specific points in time. For example, a man whose use of substances impairs his insight and motivation may not be able to fully understand his own genuine internal wishes or to work toward enacting his own personal choices. A parent who is immensely concerned about a seriously ill child may make decisions out of desperation. Similarly, an individual who is approached by his or her teacher, employer, nursing home director, longtime personal physician, military superior, or prison warden to participate in research may not feel able to refuse. A poor person may have such need for the financial compensation associated with a study that the level of risk seems irrelevant. Finally, an elderly, ethnic minority person without health insurance may feel that he or she has few options when interacting with a clinical investigator who offers health care as part of a protocol "package." Under most circumstances, the criterion of "voluntarism" is superficially fulfilled by the absence of overt coercive influences. ...such problems associated with autonomy provide further reason for the absolute integrity of investigators as a precondition for ethical human research. [10]

In light of these challenges, careful informed consent procedures will foster thorough, but not burdensome, information-sharing; allow for assessment and verification of adequate decisional capacity; and promote the voluntariness and autonomy of the participant.

Confidentiality, another safeguard important to the conduct of ethical research, is a privilege in which the personal information of a research participant and data gathered about a participant through observation and protocol procedures are protected – during the conduct of the protocol and the handling and analysis of the data and in future publications or other forms of disclosure. In most research projects, data will be confidentially encoded and not traceable to a specific individual unless the participant has specially consented to this. In recent years, with the Health Insurance Portability and Accountability Act (HIPAA) Privacy Rule gaining so much importance in clinical care, the restrictions surrounding confidentiality in research have grown even more rigorous than in the past. Concerns about confidentiality have indeed become an insurmountable barrier for certain kinds of research that pose no other risk than the potential for psychosocial harm, should a confidentiality breach occur.

Managing conflicts of interest is a safeguard that has gained prominence and attention in the broad societal dialogue about human research ethics. Threats to investigator integrity emerge from conflicts of interest, defined as motivations or situations in which the professional's ability to "observe, judge, and act according to the moral requirements of their role are, or will be, compromised" [11]. Different approaches to managing such conflicts exist, including role separation, oversight, and financial limits [12]. Such measures are less able to address non-monetized conflicts, such as the investigator's desire for rapid academic promotion or enhanced reputation. For this reason, the investigator's fundamental professionalism is perhaps the most critical safeguard of all.

Academic livelihood rests on the publication of research. The publication of clinical research findings in peer-reviewed journals, for example, is widely accepted as the basis for treatment decisions and for driving public and private healthcare policy, not to mention for public discourse and sustained academic careers. Clinical research has become increasingly complex – studies commonly involve different specialists; trials often involve various geographic sites; and as a by-product, multiple authorship is a widespread academic and intellectual issue. Increases in named authors naturally generate concerns over who has rightfully fulfilled the criteria for true authors.

As a way to clarify standards and minimize conflicts, the International Committee of Medical Journal Editors constructed the following definition of authorship on four criteria:

- Substantial contributions to the conception or design of the work; or the acquisition, analysis, or interpretation of data for the work; AND
- Drafting the work or revising it critically for important intellectual content; AND
- Final approval of the version to be published; AND
- Agreement to be accountable for all aspects of the work in ensuring that questions related to the accuracy or integrity of any part of the work are appropriately investigated and resolved [13].

This definition implies that authorship credit is not based on mere participation in research, whether in the laboratory, hospital, or community. Contributors who do not meet the authorship requirements are usually noted in the acknowledgements section or contributors' byline.

Although the vast majority of the literature promotes a rigorous application of the ICMJE criteria, some suggest that the ICMJE definition may be impractical in implementation. Others oppose the definition on conceptual grounds, raising concerns over the logic and ethics surrounding the definition. In general, the balance between effort and contribution, together with accountability, composes rightful authorship [14]. The first two components of the ICMJE criteria are concerned about the actual work and sufficient participation in it so as to allow the fulfillment of the last component, which ensures accountability and allows the assumption of public responsibility of the work.

Professional misconduct in research has been defined by the US Office of Research Integrity (ORI) to have three possible forms. One is the fabrication or creation of nonexistent data or results, which can take place in the context of proposing, performing, or reviewing research. A second form of research misconduct is the falsification or alteration of data or results in such a way that the research is not accurately stated. The last type of behavior is plagiarism, the use of someone else's ideas, results, or words without giving appropriate credit. The ORI explicitly states that misconduct does not include honest mistakes or differences of opinion. Misbehavior in research is a serious issue, one that threatens the integrity of science and undermines public trust in the whole of the scientific enterprise.

Clinical Training

Medical students and residents encounter many ethical challenges on their path to becoming independent physicians. Gaining the knowledge and skills needed to be a good doctor – a professional who serves others with competence, kindness, and compassion – is balanced against the reality that the trainee begins without sufficient knowledge and skill and must learn "with" and "through" patients. In practice, trainees often carry immense responsibilities for seriously ill individuals while acquiring greater competence, and trainees may become distressed and exhausted. Many are concerned that clinical training may inevitably produce "compassion fatigue" and diminished empathy among early-career physicians because of the burdens they shoulder, often alone and without sufficient supervision or support.

In the 1980s, several leaders in medicine assembled a list of core clinical ethics skills that were believed to be a minimally necessary set of skills which a competent physician must possess. The findings of this conference were published in the *New England Journal of Medicine* [15], and seven key skills, that is, competencies that a "minimal basic curriculum" would instill, were defined. Some of these competencies were broad, such as "the ability to identify the moral aspects of medical practice" and "ability to obtain valid consent or valid refusal of treatment," while others very clearly reflected the most salient ethical controversies at the time, for example, "knowledge of how to proceed if a patient is only partially competent or incompetent to consent to or refuse treatment," "knowledge of how to proceed if a patient refuses treatment," and "knowledge of the moral aspects of the care of patients with a poor prognosis, including patients who are terminally ill."

This early work foreshadowed the new competency movement in American medicine. Ethics and professionalism, together, have more recently been defined as a core "competence" for physicians and physicians-in-training. Trainees often encounter ethical dilemmas for which they feel unprepared, and they perceive ethics and professionalism education as important throughout a career in medicine [16–28]. The Association of American Medical Colleges has designated key learning objectives for medical student education, stating that it must prepare physicians who are altruistic, knowledgeable, skillful, and dutiful. With its robust "milestones" project, the Accreditation Council for Graduate Medical Education (ACGME) has recently implemented clearer and more rigorous expectations for residency programs regarding the evaluation of resident competence with respect to clinical ethics skills and evidence of professionalism. The ACGME mandated that, beginning in 2007, residents demonstrate "a commitment to carrying out professional responsibilities and an adherence to ethical principles" and anchored this expectation in behaviors and attitudes, including the following [29]:

- Compassion, integrity, and respect for others
- Responsiveness to patient needs that supersedes self-interest
- Respect for patient privacy and autonomy
- Accountability to patients, society, and the profession
- Sensitivity and responsiveness to a diverse patient population, including but not limited to diversity in gender, age, culture, race, religion, disabilities, and sexual orientation

The capacity to provide culturally attuned and sensitive care is also a newly recognized fundamental commitment in clinical medicine, and many efforts to define and operationalize this concept are underway (see chapter "Multicultural and Ethical Considerations in American Medicine").

Empirical studies of the views of trainees regarding ethics and professionalism education suggest the critical importance of role models and explicit and positive attention to ethics issues that otherwise become implicitly and negatively dealt with in the "hidden curriculum" [28, 30, 31]. Medical students and residents may make mistakes, and this situation generates anguish as well as real life "tests" of character and ethics. Medical students and residents observe unethical behavior routinely, and data indicate that they encounter burnout, mistreatment, and abuse commonly during training [32–36]. Studies engaging trainees have shown that ethics teaching that occurs in real time and in clinical context is especially valued, whereas educational methods that are seen as disconnected and not attuned to the ecology of clinical practice are not seen as worthwhile [16, 28].

Goals and objectives for ethics training in medicine should, in our view, be seen in the context of the natural progression of the identity of the physician (Table 4.2). Early in clinical training, the learner should be able to define and use ethics terms accurately and to identify values-laden aspects and ethical considerations present in a clinical care situation. For example, the student should recognize the ethical concerns that arise when a student is misrepresented as "a doctor" to patients in training settings. The physician-in-training should be able to demonstrate the ability to apply ethics principles in understanding and selecting among different ethically sound approaches to clinical care situations. The learner should also know how to recognize his or her own limits and, in response, to seek supervision and additional information, including relevant clinical and legal information and ethics guidelines. The physician-in-training should be able to use these resources and empirical evidence in clarifying ethical questions. Students should also be able to observe and characterize a clinical interaction and then to identify how factors in the interaction may affect the ethical dimensions of the patient's care.

Over time, the physician-in-training should be able to describe his or her training experiences within the context of professional attitudes, values, and ethics. As the early-career physician progresses, he or she should be able to assess more sophisticated, complex clinical care situations in light of clinical, ethical, psychosocial, and legal issues; to demonstrate appropriate self-directed learning and growth in ethics and professionalism; and to apply formal ethical decision-making models to ethically complex situations. Finally, in preparation for the transition to independent clinical practice, learners should be able to demonstrate their ability to perform key ethically important clinical tasks, such as obtaining informed consent or refusal for care, safeguarding confidentiality, and addressing stigmatizing health issues in a manner that reflects sensitivity, demonstrates awareness of ethical complexities present in the situation, and fulfills accepted standards of care. The independent physician, further, will show the capacity to identify a course of action that employs advanced clinical ethics problem-resolution techniques and to reflect upon his or her professional training experiences, to characterize how one's value system may influence one's clinical practices, and to safeguard against one's personal biases.

Table 4.2 Recommendations for ethics teaching in clinical training

Design curricula that address clinically relevant issues in mental health ethics including confidentiality, informed consent, decisional capacity, and end of life care
Develop special events that highlight the importance and value of ethics, e.g., grand rounds, invited visiting professors, and evidence-based ethics research presentations
Create diverse contexts for learning and self-reflection and draw out the ethical meaning within routine clinical situations
Find ways to provide additional educational opportunities for trainees who have greater interest in ethics topics and skills
Respectfully and sensitively guide trainees in identifying their own responses and defenses in relation to clinical ethical issues
Provide access to ethics resources and encourage the use of colleagues, supervisors, and expert consultants in addressing ethically complex situations
Encourage faculty mentors with an interest in ethics to obtain formal training and provide time and resources to support ethics teaching for trainees
Include ethics knowledge and skill and professional attitudes in the formal evaluation of trainees
Help trainees as they deal constructively with their own limitations and errors; without losing sight of clinical competence standards, work with trainees in seeing mistakes and bad outcome situations as unfortunate and as offering formative lessons
Seek opportunities for trainees to discuss the stresses of training and their impact upon their patient care activities, including ethically important decision-making
Strategies for implementing ethics in clinical supervision include:
Help the resident to define the clinical aspects of the patient's case
Guide the resident in the identification of ethical issues and conflicts in the clinical situation while giving them an opportunity to describe personal thoughts and concerns relating to the case
Collaborate with the resident in gathering information and necessary clinical and ethical expertise
Explore possible responses to the clinical and ethical problems with the resident, deciding what acceptable choices exist and anticipating the outcomes of these possible decisions
Provide guidance and support as the resident implements the decision and create a context for reflection and review

Review and Reflect: Ask Yourself and Talk with Colleagues

For each of the following scenarios, ask yourself and talk with colleagues about the following questions: What ethical tensions exist in this situation? What legal obligations, if any, are present? What professionalism concepts are relevant? What are the physician or physician-in-training's next steps?

Scenario 1 A physician feels that the dress and appearance of one of her colleagues is not appropriate for a professional setting. The colleague sometimes wears the same clothes for 2 days in a row, and she also sometimes comes to work smelling of alcohol. The physician is not aware of any problems or concerns in the colleague's care of patients.

Scenario 2 A third-year medicine resident sees another physician interacting with and treating a patient in a way that seems dismissive and brusque. Later the other physician is overheard speaking with a nurse, "Yeah, I didn't need to waste too much time with the consent paperwork – the patient just signed, so I didn't have to explain anything."

Scenario 3 A medical student is preparing to perform a minor surgical procedure on a patient. Apprehensive, the patient asks the student how much experience he has in performing the procedure. The student has assisted the instructor on one occasion, but he has never actually performed the procedure. In a world-weary tone of voice, the student tells the patient, "Believe me, I have enough experience." Overhearing, the instructor pulls the student aside and asks why he deliberately misled the patient about his experience level. The student responds that another esteemed doctor in the hospital had him practice saying this line and told him to always say it when a patient is unlikely to be comfortable with the real answer.

Scenario 4 A physician learns that one of his attending physician colleagues routinely dines with one of his clinical research fellows. There is speculation around the hospital that they are dating, and recently the fellow was heard "bragging" that she is getting "a lot of publications" without having to do "any of the work!"

Scenario 5 A standardized patient gives feedback to a medical student after a practice interview. The standardized patient complements the student and specifically mentions which things the student did well. At the end of the discussion, the standardized patient mentions how much the student looks like a famous actor and suggests that they get together for drinks sometime.

Scenario 6 A patient was approached to enroll in a randomized controlled clinical trial looking for novel and improved approaches for diabetes management. Participation will entail trying a new medication regimen and attending educational sessions with other clinical trials patients. The patient agrees, saying, "Oh, I have to do it! I don't want to disappoint my doctor, and I think he will give me the best experimental treatment that there is!"

Scenario 7 A senior faculty member determined that a resident wrote prescriptions for himself using a supervisor's and colleague's credentials. During mandated inpatient treatment, the resident admitted to abusing the medication. After 9 months of monitoring, he is clean and appears to be doing very well, truly embracing the life of recovery. The resident returns to his training program and is assigned to the service of the senior faculty member.

Scenario 8 During a meeting involving residents and members of a faculty, a discussion develops about the performance of a faculty member who is not present. Some faculty members start to criticize the absent colleague for his/her methods of teaching.

Scenario 9 A senior resident attending a morning didactics session detects the scent of alcohol in the room. The lecturer is a senior clinician expert from the community. She cannot be sure about the smell and its origin, but it seems stronger when she approaches the lecturer at the end of the session.

Acknowledgments The following authors contributed to the scenarios in this chapter: Laura Weiss Roberts, M.D., M.A., Daryn Reicherter, M.D., Richard Balon, M.D., Teresita A. McCarty, M.D., Christine Moutier, M.D.

References

1. Office of the Secretary, U.S. Department of Health, Education, and Welfare. Belmont report: Ethical Principles and Guidelines for the Protection of Human Subjects of Research. The National Commission for the Protection of Human Subjects of Biomedical and Behavioral Research, April 18, 1979. Available at http://www.hhs.gov/ohrp/humansubjects/guidance/belmont.html. Accessed 22 Oct 2014.
2. U.S. Advisory Committee on Human Radiation Experiments. The Human Radiation Experiments: Final Report of the President's Advisory Committee. New York: Oxford University Press; 1996.
3. Applebaum BC, Applebaum PS, Grisso T. Competence to consent to voluntary psychiatric hospitalization: a test of a standard proposed by APA. American Psychiatric Association. Psychiatr Serv. 1998;49(9):1193–6.
4. Shamoo AE. Human Rights in reference to persons with mental illness. Account Res. 1996;4(3–4):207–16.
5. U.S. Department of Health and Human Services. Code of Federal Regulations, Title 45, Part 46, Protection of Human Subjects. Revised 15 Jan 2009. Available at http://www.hhs.gov.laneproxy.stanford.edu/ohrp/humansubjects/guidance/45cfr46.html. Accessed 22 Oct 2014.
6. Applebaum PS, Roth LH, Lidz C. The therapeutic misconception: informed consent in psychiatric research. Int J Law Psychiatry. 1982;5(3–4):319–29.
7. Dresser R. Mentally disabled research subjects. The enduring policy issues. JAMA. 1996;276(1):67–72.
8. Levine RJ. Research that could yield marketable products from human materials: the problem of informed consent. IRB. 1986;8(1):6–7.
9. National Bioethics Advisory Commission. Research involving persons with mental disorders that may affect decision making capacity. Rockville: National Bioethics Advisory Commission; 1998.
10. Roberts LW, Dyer AR. Concise guide to ethics in mental health care. Washington, DC: American Psychiatric Publishing; 2004.
11. Shimm DS, Spece Jr RG. Introduction. In: Spece Jr RG, Shimm DS, Buchanan AE, editors. Conflicts of interest in clinical practice and research. New York: Oxford University Press; 1996.
12. Korn D, Carlat D. Conflicts of interest in medical education: recommendations from the pew task force on medical conflicts of interest. JAMA. 2013;310(22):2397–8.
13. International Committee of Medical Journal Editors. Recommendations for the conduct, reporting, editing, and publication of scholarly work in medical journals. January 31, 2014. Available at http://www.icmje.org/recommendations/. Accessed 22 Oct 2014.
14. Tsao CI, Roberts LW. Authorship in scholarly manuscripts: practical considerations for resident and early career physicians. Acad Psychiatry. 2009;33(1):76–9.
15. Culver CM, Clouser KD, Gert B, et al. Basic curricular goals in medical ethics. The DeCamp report. NEJM. 1985;312:253–6.

16. Marrero IM, Bell M, Dunn L, Roberts LW. Assessing professionalism and ethics knowledge and skills: preferences of psychiatry residents. Acad Psychiatry. 2013;37:392–7.
17. Jain S, Lapid MI, Dunn LB, Roberts LW. Psychiatric residents' needs for education about informed consent, principles of ethics and professionalism, and caring for vulnerable populations: results of a multisite survey. Acad Psychiatry. 2011;35(3):184–90.
18. Jain S, Dunn L, Warner C, Roberts LW. Results of a multisite survey of U.S. psychiatry residents on education in professionalism and ethics. Acad Psychiatry. 2011;35(3):175–83.
19. Jain S, Hoop JG, Dunn LB, Roberts LW. Psychiatry residents' attitudes on ethics and professionalism: multisite survey results. Ethics Behav. 2010;20:10–20.
20. Lapid M, Moutier C, Dunn L, Green Hammond K, Roberts LW. Professionalism and ethics education on relationships and boundaries: psychiatric residents' training preferences. Acad Psychiatry. 2009;33(6):461–9.
21. Lehrmann J, Hoop JG, Green Hammond K, Roberts LW. Medical students' affirmation of ethics education. Acad Psychiatry. 2009;33(6):470–7.
22. Roberts LW, Warner TD, Dunn LB, Brody JL, Hammond KGA, Roberts BB. Shaping medical students' attitudes toward ethically important aspects of clinical research: results of a randomized, controlled educational intervention. Ethics Behav. 2007;17(1):19–50.
23. Warner TD, Geppert CMA, Massone J, Roberts LW. Views of ten chief residents on professionalism and ethics training. Ann Behav Sci Med Edu. 2006;12(1):12–20.
24. Roberts LW, Geppert CM, Warner TD, Green Hammond K, Lamberton L. Bioethics principles, informed consent, and ethical care for special populations: Curricular needs expressed by men and women physicians-in-training. Psychosomatics. 2005;46(5):440–50.
25. Roberts LW, Geppert CM, Warner TD, Green Hammond K, Heinrich T. Becoming a good doctor: perceived need for ethics training focused on practical and professional development topics. Acad Psychiatry. 2005;29(3):301–9.
26. Roberts LW, Warner TD, Green Hammond K, Brody JL, Kaminsky A, Roberts BB. Teaching medical students to discern ethical problems in human clinical research studies. Acad Med. 2005;80(10):925–30.
27. Roberts LW, Green Hammond K, Warner TW, Geppert CG. The positive role of professionalism and ethics training in medical education: a comparison of medical student and resident perspectives. Acad Psychiatry. 2004;28(3):170–82.
28. Roberts LW, et al. What and how psychiatry residents at ten training programs wish to learn about ethics. Acad Psychiatry. 1996;20(3):127–39.
29. Accreditation Council for Graduate Medical Education. Psychiatry Program Requirements. Chicago, IL: Accreditation Council for Graduate Medical Education; 2007.
30. Coverdale JH, et al. Are we teaching psychiatrists to be ethical? Acad Psychiatry. 1992;16(4):199–205.
31. Louie AK, Roberts LW, Coverdale J. The enculturation of medical students and residents. Acad Psychiatry. 2007;31(4):253–7.
32. Roberts LW. Understanding depression and distress among medical students. JAMA. 2010;304(11):1231–3.
33. Coverdale JH, Balon R, Roberts LW. Mistreatment of trainees: verbal abuse and other bullying behaviors. Acad Psychiatry. 2009;33(4):269–73.
34. Roberts LW. Hard duty. Acad Psychiatry. 2009;33(4):274–7.
35. Dyrbye LN, Thomas MR, Huntington JL, Lawson KL, Novotny PJ, Sloan JA, Shanafelt TD. Systematic review of depression, anxiety, and other indicators of psychological distress among U.S. and Canadian medical students. Acad Med. 2006;81(4):374–84.
36. Dyrbye LN, West CP, Satele D, Boone S, Tan L, Sloan J, Shanafelt TD. Burnout among U.S. medical students, residents, and early career physicians relative to the general U.S. population. Acad Med. 2014;89(3):443–51.

Recommended Reading

Beauchamp TL, Childress JF. Principles of biomedical ethics. 6th ed. New York: Oxford University
    Press; 2008.
Bloch S, Chodoff P, editors. Psychiatric ethics. Oxford: Oxford University Press; 1999.
Jonsen AR, Siegler M, Winslade WJ. Clinical ethics: A practical approach to ethical decisions in
    clinical medicine. 7th ed. New York: McGraw-Hill; 2010.
Kushe H, Singer P. A companion to bioethics. Oxford: Blackwell; 1998.

Chapter 5
Professionalism in Medicine as a Transnational and Transcultural Ethical Concept

John H. Coverdale and Lawrence B. McCullough

The ethical concept of professionalism in medicine must do a great deal of work. The concept ought to be transnational and transcultural and endure over time. The concept should also be comprehensive in scope, applying to medical practice, medical education, and biomedical research. The concept should be practical, providing a framework to guide culturally sensitive and culturally competent clinical judgment, decision-making, and behavior for practicing physicians and trainees across all specialties and subspecialties. This is a daunting set of requirements for any concept to meet.

Many physicians take for granted that the ethical concept of medicine as a profession originated in ancient Greece, in the Oath and other writings attributed to Hippocrates. There are alternative ideas about the origin [1, 2]. In fact, the concept of medicine as a profession originated in the ethical writings of two British physicians [3], the Scottish physician-ethicist John Gregory (1724–1773) and the English physician-ethicist Thomas Percival (1740–1804).

J.H. Coverdale, M.D., M.Ed. (✉)
Menninger Department of Psychiatry and Behavioral Sciences,
Baylor College of Medicine, Houston, TX, USA
e-mail: jhc@bcm.edu

L.B. McCullough, Ph.D.
Center for Medical Ethics and Health Policy,
Baylor College of Medicine, Houston, TX, USA

© Springer Science+Business Media New York 2015
L.W. Roberts, D. Reicherter (eds.), *Professionalism and Ethics in Medicine*,
DOI 10.1007/978-1-4939-1686-3_5

Historical Origins of the Ethical Concept of Medicine as a Profession

The Absence of an Ethical Concept of Medicine as a Profession in Hippocrates

Robert Baker calls the belief that the ethical concept of medicine as a profession originates in the Hippocratic Oath and other texts, the "myth of the Hippocratic footnote." This phrase captures the idea that the history of Western medical ethics is but a footnote to the Hippocratic Oath and texts [1]. Scholars such as Baker and Vivian Nutton [4] have shown that this reading does not bear close scrutiny, if only because the Oath itself did not have much of an influence on the subsequent history of medical ethics. Indeed, it largely fell out of favor during the early Christian era and was only resurrected in the nineteenth century. The Oath has taken on a symbolic value in the recent history of medical ethics.

There are two substantive reasons not to adopt the Hippocratic Oath as the source for modern professional medical ethics. The Oath contains a series of admonitions, such as the prohibitions against using a pessary to induce an abortion, sexual contact with or abuse of patients, and surgery for which no supporting reasons are given. Nowhere in the Oath or in the other Hippocratic texts do their authors set out a conceptual framework and reasoning using that framework to justify these admonitions. This failure does not meet the standards of argument-based ethics [5].

The second reason is that the Hippocratic texts are not clearly texts in professional medical ethics. This is because they are characterized by a deep and unresolved tension between the commitment to the well being of patients, on the one hand, and the physician's self-interests, on the other. It is important to recall that in ancient Greece, there was no uniform medical education, no licensure, and no third-party payers but, instead, a genuine market in which physicians competed fiercely with other practitioners, both secular and sacred, for the small market of the sick who could afford their fees, with no regulation by the state or effective self-regulation by associations of physicians (the royal colleges). Failure to succeed in this Darwinian market meant economic ruin.

Success in the market required maintenance of trust. The prohibition against sexual contact in the Oath could be interpreted as a promise that the women and men, both free and slave, of a paying customer's household will be safe, an excellent marketing tool to promote trust. This prohibition can also be read as an expression of prohibited boundary crossing on the basis of a professional obligation to prevent harm to those over whom one has power. The problem is that we do not know how to resolve this tension given the lack of a clear conceptual framework and argument based on it.

The subsequent history of Western medicine has shown that the deep tension in the Hippocratic texts between a life of service to the sick and entrepreneurial self-interest was resolved more in the direction of entrepreneurial self-interest than in the direction of a life of service to the sick [4]. The latter commitment was sustained mostly in religious communities and in Christian, Jewish, and Islamic medical ethics. In secular medical ethics, which emerged during the Renaissance, the virtue of prudence comes to great prominence. This is a virtue that instructs physicians to identify their legitimate self-interests. Prudence becomes central to a series of books on medical ethics with the title *Medicus Politicus*, or the politic doctor [6]. This tradition culminated in the *Medicus Politicus* of the German physician Friedrich Hoffmann. Hoffmann called for physicians to base their practice on enlightened self-interest, in an attempt to rein in the excesses of entrepreneurial practice but not to reform it.

The modern ethical concept of medicine as a profession did not originate in ancient Greece or Renaissance Europe. Its origin is much more recent, in the writings of Gregory and Percival [3]. These physicians wrote their medical ethics in response to what they took to be the morally corrosive aspects of entrepreneurial, self-interested medicine. They self-consciously used medical ethics to reform clinical practice and research from an entrepreneurial, marketplace model into a professional model.

Eighteenth-century British medicine (including British medicine in the American colonies) was characterized by intense competition in an unforgiving marketplace of promoting and selling medical services to the well-to-do, who paid the piper and therefore called the tune. There was no uniform pathway of education to become a physician, surgeon, or apothecary and there was a surfeit of practitioners. There were almost as many concepts of health and disease, and remedies for the latter, as there were practitioners. In order to win the favor of rich patients, physicians hired manners coaches to teach them how to speak, dress, and comport themselves in the presence of their social and political betters. Being well mannered was crucial for bridging the class difference between physicians, who mainly came from the middle classes, and the landed aristocracy and wealthy merchants, who were the social and political superiors of physicians. Patients worried about the man of false manners, that is, the physician who used good manners to insinuate himself into the houses of the rich, to take advantage of them. This included sexual advantage, resulting in worries by rich men about the sexual predations of doctors on their wives and daughters. Gregory and Percival were also concerned about the lack of scientific and clinical competence and rampant self-interest that distorted clinical judgment, practice, and research [4].

Gregory on the Ethical Concept of Medicine as a Profession

Gregory, especially, was concerned that the lack of scientific competence and unbridled self-interest made the already perilous condition of the sick even more perilous. The sick could not intellectually trust physicians to know what they were doing and could not morally trust physicians to put the interests of the sick rather than physicians' own interest first. Gregory's view was that this was a terrible

Table 5.1 Ethical concept of medicine as a profession [3]

The physician should become and remain scientifically and clinically competent.
Based on the scientific method of Francis Bacon (1561–1626), a nascent form of evidence-based medicine
The physician should commit to the protection and promotion of the health-related interests of the patient as the physician's primary concern and motivation.
The physician's self-interests are blunted by professional virtues and obligations to the patient.
Physicians should maintain, strengthen, and pass on medicine to future physicians and patients as a public trust, not merchant guild.

experience for the sick. His remarkable insight was to see that the plight of the sick had unacceptable moral implications for physicians who had any capacity for compassion. His remedy was to reform medicine into a profession, using the tools of medical ethics and philosophy of medicine.

Gregory based his medical ethics on David Hume's principle of sympathy [4]. Sympathy is a natural capacity of each morally well-formed human being to enter into and experience the sufferings of others and to be motivated routinely to relieve and prevent such suffering. Gregory thought that the plight of the sick created by intellectual and moral distrust, both well-to-do and worthy poor, was not acceptable. Moreover, Gregory was very concerned that the entrepreneurial, self-interested practice of medicine introduced biases that disabled clinical judgment and decision-making, calling into question the very competence of physicians. Gregory addressed the problem of competence by appealing to the philosophy of science and medicine of Francis Bacon (1561–1626). Bacon called for medicine to be based on "experience," that is, the rigorously collected and described results of natural and designed experiments. In effect, Bacon called for medicine to become evidence based, a call that medicine is now answering five centuries after it was issued.

Before Gregory, physicians routinely used the word *profession* to describe themselves. They used this word in a self-interested way, to distinguish themselves from practitioners who had not attended a university and received a "regular" education (a dubious claim on its face, given the absence of a stable medical curriculum) and that their competitors – surgeons, apothecaries, and "irregular" practitioners – had not done so and were therefore inferior practitioners [4]. Gregory set out to give *profession* intellectual and moral content. In doing so, he put in place the first two of the three components that constitute the ethical concept of medicine as a profession (Table 5.1).

The first component of the ethical concept of medicine as a profession is that physicians should become and remain scientifically and clinically competent. In contemporary terms, this means that physicians should practice according to the intellectual and clinical discipline of evidence-based medicine, also called the deliberative practice of medicine. When physicians routinely do so, they justifiably invite the sick to trust them intellectually, to know what they are saying and doing. The scientific and clinical competence of physicians is confined to health, understood in biopsychosocial terms [7]. Physicians set themselves up for entirely preventable ethical conflict when they fail to stay within the bounds of their professional expertise and authority.

The second component of the ethical concept of medicine as a profession is that physicians should commit themselves to the protection and promotion of the health-related interests of the sick as their primary concern and motivation, keeping self-interest systematically secondary. Gregory based this second component on the principle of sympathy, or fellow feeling, of his contemporary David Hume (1711–1776) [4].

In his *Lectures,* Gregory set out his general account of sympathy, which he then deployed to consider a wide range of clinical topics (a list that essentially anticipated the entire agenda of clinical ethics save for organizational ethics).

> I come now to mention the moral qualities peculiarly required in the character of a physician. The chief of these is humanity; that sensibility of heart which makes us feel for the distresses of our fellow-creatures, and which, of consequence, incites us in the most powerful manner to relieve them. Sympathy produces an anxious attention to a thousand little circumstances that may tend to relieve the patient; an attention which money can never purchase: hence the inexpressible comfort of having a friend for a physician. Sympathy naturally engages the affection and confidence of a patient, which, in many cases, is of the utmost consequence to his recovery. If the physician possesses gentleness of manners, and a compassionate heart, and what Shakespeare so emphatically calls "the milk of human kindness," the patient feels his approach like that of a guardian angel ministering to his relief: while every visit of a physician who is unfeeling, and rough in his manners, makes his heart sink within him, as at the presence of one, who comes to pronounce his doom. Men of the most compassionate tempers, by being daily conversant with scenes of distress, acquire in process of time that composure and firmness of mind so necessary in the practice of physick. They can feel whatever is amiable in pity, without suffering it to enervate or unman them. Such physicians as are callous to sentiments of humanity, treat this sympathy with ridicule, and represent it either as hypocrisy, or as the indication of a feeble mind. That sympathy is often affected, I am afraid is true. But this affectation may be easily seen through. Real sympathy is never ostentatious; on the contrary, it rather strives to conceal itself. But, what most effectually detects this hypocrisy, is a physician's different manner of behaving to people in high and people in low life; to those who reward him handsomely, and those who have not the means to do it. A generous and elevated mind is even more shy in expressing sympathy with those of high rank, than with those in humbler life; being jealous of the unworthy construction so usually annexed to it. – The insinuation that a compassionate and feeling heart is commonly accompanied with a weak understanding and a feeble mind, is malignant and false. Experience demonstrates, that a gentle and humane temper, so far from being inconsistent with vigour of mind, is its usual attendant; and that rough and blustering manners generally accompany a weak understanding and a mean soul, and are indeed frequently affected by men void of magnanimity and personal courage, ['in order' added in errata] to conceal their natural defects. ([8], pp. 19–21)

The first two components of the ethical concept of fiduciary professionalism are expressed in the bedrock professional virtue of integrity. The professional virtue of integrity obligates physicians to practice medicine, conduct research, and teach to standards of intellectual excellence (the first component of the concept of fiduciary professionalism) and to standards of moral excellence (the second component of the concept of fiduciary professionalism).

Gregory gestured in the direction of the third component of the ethical concept of medicine as a profession when he excoriated the "corporation spirit" of the organized medicine of his own day, i.e., the royal colleges operating under the auspices of a royal charter.

> I hope I have advanced no opinions in these Lectures that tend to lessen the dignity of a profession which has always been considered as most honourable and important. But, I apprehend, this dignity is not to be supported by a narrow, selfish, corporation-spirit; by self-importance; by a formality in dress and manners, or by an affectation of mystery. The true dignity of physic is to be maintained by the superior learning and abilities of those who profess it, by the liberal manners of gentlemen; and by that openness and candour, which disdain all artifice, which invite to a free enquiry, and thus boldly bid defiance to all that illiberal ridicule and abuse, to which medicine has been so much and so long exposed. ([8], pp. 236–237)

The royal colleges were, essentially, merchant guilds that existed and conducted themselves primarily for the sake of the interests of their members in gaining and holding market share. The self-interested nature of the royal colleges was reflected in their moral "statutes," or rules of conduct. These included prohibitions against attacking brother physicians in public, so as not to injure the profession, that is, the interests of guild members in presenting an attractive public face to their potential customers among the well-to-do [4].

Percival on the Ethical Concept of Medicine as a Profession

Percival should be given the credit for picking up on Gregory's gesture and then explicitly expressing it in conceptual terms [3]. Percival sets out the third component of the ethical concept of medicine as a profession in his discussion of the ethics of when a physician or surgeon should retire from practice. He provides insightful analysis of the intellectual skills such as an acute memory and the ability to reason by analogy from present to past cases and, for surgeons, skills such as "quickness of eye-sight, delicacy of touch, and steadiness of hand, which are essential to the skillful performance of operations" ([9], p. 52). This passage is especially moving in light of the fact that Percival by then had become blind and retired from medical practice, thus following and exemplifying his argument. He concludes:

> Let both the physician and surgeon never forget, that their professions are public trusts, properly rendered lucrative whilst they fulfil them; but which they are bound, by honour and probity, to relinquish, as soon as they find themselves unequal to their adequate and faithful execution. ([9], p. 52)

Gregory and Percival were the first in the history of Western medical ethics to consistently use the word *patient* rather than the phrase *the sick* – for the Latin, *aegrotus*, which is used in previous texts – and in so doing, they drew an important implication from the ethical concept of medicine as a profession. Until medicine became a profession, a process that started with Gregory and Percival and still has a long way to go if critics such as Rothman are correct [10], there were no physicians, only practitioners of various kinds. Routinely fulfilling the three commitments required by the concept of medicine as a profession turns medical practitioners into professional physicians. In other words, the profession of medicine is not a given that comes down to us from the stylus of Hippocrates robustly intact over the centuries. Rather, the profession of medicine exists as a function of the collective clinical judgments, decisions, and behaviors of physicians. External entities such as payers do not create the profession of medicine, and they cannot destroy or injure it. Physicians are fully in charge of the profession of medicine and should hold themselves accountable for maintaining it [11].

When there are professional physicians, the sick become patients. They can and should trust professional physicians both intellectually and morally. The older, contractual relationship of the sick and hired practitioners becomes replaced with a physician-patient relationship as a fiduciary relationship of protection and promotion of the patient's and research subject's health-related interests.

Implications for Medical Practice, Research, and Education

The first component of the ethical concept of medicine as a profession requires medical practice, research, and education to be based on the deliberative practice of medicine, that is, submitting to the discipline of evidence-based reasoning. Physicians and other healthcare professionals who accept this discipline exhibit intellectual integrity that justifies the trust of patients, payers, healthcare organizations, and society.

As a matter of intellectual integrity, healthcare professionals should not assert the autonomy to practice as they prefer but only the autonomy to practice as they should. Organizational leaders should not accept the first expression of autonomy but only the second. The commitment to evidence-based practice is also essential for the successful cooperation of the multiple disciplines that contribute to excellent medical care.

The second component of the ethical concept of medicine as a profession requires healthcare professionals to put the health-related interests of patients first and keep self-interest systematically secondary. The professional virtue of self-sacrifice requires healthcare professionals to responsibly manage conflicts of interest and conflicts of commitment. Conflicts of interest occur when professional responsibility to patients comes into conflict with the clinician's individual self-interest. Conflicts of commitment occur when professional responsibility comes into conflict with obligations that the clinician holds outside of professional practice, such as to family members.

Conflicts of interest should be responsibly managed by distinguishing between legitimate and mere self-interest. Legitimate self-interest concerns the necessary and sufficient conditions for excellent clinical practice, such as time to read, improve clinical skills, and rest. Legitimate self-interests also include engagement in activities outside of healthcare that gives one's overall life meaning and purpose. Mere self-interests are those forms of self-interest not in these two categories. The professional virtue of self-sacrifice requires that conflicts between professional responsibility and mere self-interest always be resolved in favor of professional responsibility. The professional virtue of self-sacrifice becomes tyrannical if it does not allow for the protection of legitimate self-interest, under a crucial constraint: patients' clinical needs must be met. Thus, the need to respond to a medical psychiatric emergency always overrides legitimate self-interests. The professional virtue of self-sacrifice does not rule out setting limits on one's practice on the basis of legitimate self-interest, for example, reducing one's clinical hours to engage in meaningful activities outside of clinical practice, understanding that loss of income will result. Taking time for such activities promotes maturity and wisdom, which are essential in routine medical practice.

Conflicts of commitment are ethically and personally more challenging, because one cannot release oneself from obligations to others: either others must release one from the obligations or one must make a very compelling case that such obligations should be violated. Once again, responding to medical emergencies meets this test. In all other clinical circumstances, organizational policy and practice should minimize conflicts of commitment. For example, a clinician who is a single parent of a child with special needs may need to have different call schedule than a clinician who is unpartnered and without children or parents requiring care. Successful organizational management of the variation in conflicts of commitment requires transparency by organizational leaders and tolerance by professional staff. "Gaming the system" to advance mere self-interest rather than fulfillment of commitments should be prohibited.

The professional virtue of compassion requires clinicians to recognize and prevent pain, distress, and suffering in patients and to respond rapidly and effectively when patients do experience pain, distress, and suffering by effectively managing them. Healthcare professionals must become and remain empathically attuned to their patients in order to fulfill the professional obligations generated by the professional virtue of compassion. The professional virtue of self-effacement requires clinicians to identity social and cultural differences with patients that are clinically irrelevant and not allow awareness of such differences to bias clinical judgment, decision-making, and practice. For example, failure to recognize and discipline sexual attraction to a patient can result in impermissible boundary crossings that biopsychosocially injure patients [12].

The professional virtue of self-effacement prevents feelings that can unhinge clinical judgment [13]. Some of these feelings are appropriate and expectable, for example, the compassion-generated foreboding that arises when one must discharge a homeless patient back to the street without adequate social supports. Some of these feelings are inappropriate, such as personal repugnance to patients who are very unkempt and who emit offensive body odors. Adherence to the requirements of the professional virtues keeps the healthcare professional focused on the patient's needs and not his or her own.

The professional virtues bring to prominence the ethical dimension of a core component of good healthcare. Clinicians should work assiduously to monitor their personality, to develop maturity and wisdom, to engage in the felt world of patients without becoming unhinged, and to be consistently thoughtful in every patient encounter. Mindfulness and sensitivity guide these well-known aspects of healthcare. The professional virtues provide their justification, an often-underappreciated implication of the ethical concept of medicine as a profession.

Biomedical research involving human subjects has two components: scientific and ethical integrity; combined, they protect human subjects. Scientific integrity flows directly from the first component of the ethical concept of medicine as profession and ethical integrity from its second component. This has a major implication for research ethics: clinical investigators and team members in biomedical research have a professional responsibility to offer research only when it is designed and conducted to standards of scientific excellence and only when its risks are justified by its expected benefit. The informed consent process must convey this information in a meaningful fashion and ensure a voluntary decision about enrollment. On this approach, the ethics of research work hand in glove with the ethics of clinical practice.

A crucial aspect of professional education and training is the formation of the professional persona, which is well understood in psychiatry and the mental health professions. The formation of the professional persona should be understood in explicitly ethical terms: the commitment to the three components of the ethical concept of medicine as a profession and the professional virtues of integrity, self-sacrifice, compassion, and self-effacement. Health professions educators should role commitment to the three components of professionalism and the four professional virtues. The formal, and especially the informal or "hidden," curriculum should be routinely critically appraised for its support of ethically guided professional formation.

John Gregory's and Thomas Percival's original eighteenth-century ethical concept of medicine as a profession applies transnationally and transculturally because its three components are not limited to Western culture. Their concept therefore applies to all levels of medical practice, research, and education today. The concept also provides an everyday, practical framework for the provision of care that is culturally sensitive and culturally competent because it will be professional medical care. The concept obligated all healthcare professionals to learn and practice according to the standards of evidence-based reasoning. Moreover, the professional virtues of integrity, compassion, self-effacement, self-sacrifice, and courage direct the attention of clinicians, health professions educators, and biomedical investigators to the interests and needs of patients and away from personal needs. These are professional virtues that should be actively cultivated in order to practice to standards of intellectual and moral excellence.

Review and Reflect. Ask Yourself and Talk with Colleagues

For each of the following scenarios, ask yourself and talk with colleagues about the following questions: What ethical tensions exist in this situation? What legal obligations, if any, are present? What key concepts related to professionalism should be considered? What are the clinician's next steps?

Scenario 1 A physician notices on her schedule that she will be seeing the mother of her best friend from childhood for an initial patient visit. After the physician enters the examination room, the patient begins talking about all the fun times the physician and the patient's daughter had as children and teenagers. Next, she proceeds to describe her chronic pain issues and asks for a prescription for narcotic medications. Upon chart review, the physician notes that the patient has not had an adequate work-up for her symptoms and that she has received multiple opiate prescriptions from multiple physicians within the same practice for several years. The patient notes that she is a very busy person with full-time employment, and, therefore, she is uninterested in proceeding with a comprehensive work-up. In addition, she states she would like to be pain-free for her daughter's wedding in a month.

Scenario 2 A group of military medics are working as operating room technicians in a small military community hospital. Several are notified that they will be deploying on an overseas mission, where they will be expected to care for combat casualties in support hospitals or on forward surgical teams. In preparation for the deployment, the medics decide that they would like to become proficient in suturing. One of the medics approaches a surgeon about providing instruction in suturing during an active surgical case.

Scenario 3 A medical school dean for admissions notices that applicants from particular ethnic backgrounds are more likely to present gifts to her and the admissions staff, both during the application process and also once they are accepted to medical school. She feels generally uncomfortable about these gifts but also feels she may be rude if she turns down gifts, especially in particular cultures. The dean wonders whether she should continue to accept gifts?

Scenario 4 A medical assistant in a very busy clinic with a perpetual smile and high energy, is popular with the patients and the staff, and everyone appreciates her. Her weight noticeably fluctuates, and her teeth are severely decaying. She also has developed a facial tic. She, however, continues to do excellent work. She dresses according to the dress code, always wears her name badge, and consistently receives rave reviews on quality surveys. Although she never exceeds her allotted breaks at work, she spends them in the restroom. One weekend, a physician in the clinic sees her in a part of town where crystal methamphetamine dealers congregate.

Scenario 5 A clinician's direct supervisor is a highly esteemed senior faculty member. He is terrific to work within most ways but occasionally does not come to work.

Everyone in the office knows not to ask or say much. When the clinician has asked him if he is okay, he offers a different medical problem each time in explanation. Recently, he seems to be leaving work early and treating patients in an abrupt manner, not noted in the past.

Scenario 6 A physician is asked by his childhood friend to provide a prescription for a medication used to treat a sexually transmitted infection. The friend lives in another city. He does not want to go to his usual doctor because he is embarrassed. He also does not want documentation of the request to go into his medical record "back home."

Scenario 7 The director of an academic medical clinic supervises five physicians. In this role, his input is critical in hiring, firing, and promotions. He lives with a man in a committed but closeted relationship. When a physician in the clinic has dinner at their house, the director confides that he has hired his partner to work in the clinic and asks her to keep the information to herself. He received approval to hire his partner as a clinical assistant professor, the same level as she and the other doctors in the clinic. Nobody else knows that the men are romantic partners.

Scenario 8 A patient requests documentation of disability during pregnancy so that she can stop working but still receive income from her job. She states, "I can't walk because my legs are so swollen. I am very uncomfortable at work. I have to go to the bathroom all the time and it makes it hard to work." The complaints are subjective, and the doctor does not have clinical indications of physical disability that would prevent the patient from working.

Scenario 9 At the table in the hospital cafeteria, a physician notices two colleagues who are loudly discussing one of the well-known local celebrities. The celebrity patient had just been admitted to the hospital. No mention is made of specific clinical issues.

Acknowledgments The following authors contributed to the scenarios in this chapter: Laura Weiss Roberts, M.D., M.A., Daryn Reicherter, M.D., Richard Balon, M.D., Jodi K. Casados, M.D., Steven B. McCann, M.D., Lawrence M. McGlynn, M.D., Christine Moutier, M.D., Christopher Warner, M.D., LTC.

References

1. Baker RB. Deciphering Percival's code. In: Baker R, Porter D, Porter R, editors. The codification of medical morality: historical and philosophical studies of the formalization of western medical morality in the eighteenth and nineteenth centuries, Medical ethics and etiquette in the eighteenth century, vol. 1. Dordrecht: Kluwer; 1993. p. 179–211.
2. Nutton V. The discourses of European practitioners in the tradition of the Hippocratic texts. In: Baker RB, McCullough LB, editors. The Cambridge world history of medical ethics. New York: Cambridge University Press; 2009. p. 359–62.

3. McCullough LB. The ethical concept of medicine as a profession: its origins in modern medical ethics and implications for physicians. In: Kenny N, Shelton W, editors. Lost virtue: professional character development in medical education. New York: Elsevier; 2006. p. 17–27.
4. McCullough LB. John Gregory and the invention of professional medical ethics and the profession of medicine. Dordrecht: Kluwer; 1998.
5. McCullough LB, Coverdale JH, Chervenak FA. Argument-based ethics: a formal tool for critically appraising the normative medical ethics literature. Am J Obstet Gynecol. 2004;191: 1097–102.
6. Lindemann M. The discourses of practitioners in eighteenth-century France and Germany. In: Baker RB, McCullough LB, editors. The Cambridge world history of medical ethics. New York: Cambridge University Press; 2009. p. 391–402.
7. Engel G. The need for a new medical model: a challenge for biomedicine. Science. 1977;196:129–36. Reproduced in Holistic Med 1989;4:37–53.
8. Gregory J. Lectures on the duties and qualifications of a physician. London: W. Strahan and T. Cadell; 1772. Reprinted in McCullough LB, editor. John Gregory's writings on medical ethics and philosophy of medicine. Dordrecht: Kluwer, 1998. p. 161–245.
9. Percival T. Medical ethics: or a code of institutes and precepts, adapted to the professional conduct of physicians and surgeons. London: J. Johnson & R. Bickerstaff; 1803.
10. Rothman DJ. Medical professionalism – focusing on the real issues. N Engl J Med. 2000;342:1284–6.
11. McCullough LB. An ethical framework for the responsible leadership of accountable care organizations. Am J Med Qual. 2012;27(3):189–94.
12. McCullough LB, Chervenak FA, Coverdale JH. Ethically justified guidelines for defining sexual boundaries between obstetrician-gynecologists and their patients. Am J Obstet Gynecol. 1996;175:496–500.
13. McCullough LB, Coverdale JH, Chervenak FA. Ethical challenges of decision making with pregnant patients who have schizophrenia. Am J Obstet Gynecol. 2002;187:696–702.

Recommended Reading

Baker RB, McCullough LB, editors. The Cambridge world history of medical ethics. Cambridge: Cambridge University Press; 2008.
Jonsen AR. Short history of medical ethics. New York: Oxford University Press; 2008.
Percival T. Medical ethics: Or a code of institutes and precepts, adapted to the professional conduct of physicians and surgeons. London: J. Johnson & R. Bickerstaff; 1803.

Part II
Questions and Answers

Chapter 6
Questions with Narrative Answers

Laura Weiss Roberts and Daryn Reicherter

This chapter contains questions from across medical disciplines. Each question is followed by five possible answers, a narrative explanation of the question, and the correct answer. The narrative explanations are intended to help the learner understand applications of the fundamental principles of professionalism and ethics in medicine set forth in Part I. The learner may refer back to the relevant chapter in Part I for the conceptual framework.

1. Decisional capacity is understood to have four necessary elements. Which of the following is the correct set of four elements?

   A. To appreciate, to communicate, to reason, and to understand.
   B. To assent, to understand, to translate, and to verify.
   C. To communicate, to articulate, to reason, and to translate.
   D. To deduce, to reason, to speak, and to verify.
   E. To reason, to speak, to indicate, and to understand.

   In 1998, Appelbaum and Grisso proposed a model for decisional capacity with four essential elements: (1) the ability to communicate a preference,

---

Contributing authors: Laura Weiss Roberts, M.D., M.A., Daryn Reicherter, M.D., John H. Coverdale, M.D., M.Ed., Kristi R. Estabrook, M.D., Cynthia M. A. Geppert, M.D., M.P.H., Ph.D., Shaili Jain, M.D., Sermsak Lolak, M.D., Celeste Lopez, M.D., Lawrence McCullough, Ph.D., Lawrence M. McGlynn, M.D., Christine Moutier, M.D., Joshua Reiher, M.D., Richard Shaw, M.D., Christopher Warner, M.D., LTC

L.W. Roberts, M.D., M.A. (✉) • D. Reicherter, M.D.
Department of Psychiatry and Behavioral Sciences,
Stanford University School of Medicine, Stanford, CA, USA
e-mail: RobertsL@stanford.edu

© Springer Science+Business Media New York 2015
L.W. Roberts, D. Reicherter (eds.), *Professionalism and Ethics in Medicine*,
DOI 10.1007/978-1-4939-1686-3_6

(2) the ability to understand, (3) the ability to reason, and (4) the ability to appreciate the nature of the decision and its ramifications. This model has become the fundamental standard clinically, legally, and ethically in the United States. Answer: A

2. A 17-year-old Vietnamese refugee presents to a gastrointestinal specialist with diarrhea, nausea, and vague complaints of abdominal pain that are not well understood by her primary care doctor. She appears very anxious. She says that her mother took her to a traditional healer earlier that day. She has deep, red marks on her forehead and forearms and large circular bruises on her back. What is the responsibility of the specialist?

A. Report the case to Child Protective Services.
B. Remove the girl from her parents.
C. Find out more about the marks to rule out any child mistreatment.
D. Ignore the marks and treat the gastrointestinal symptoms.
E. Report the traditional healer to the police.

"Coining" and "cupping" are common folk treatments for somatic symptoms in people from South East Asia. "Coining" is a benign folk remedy that treats various ailments by using the edge of a coin or similar object to scrape or "scratch" the skin. "Cupping" is an ancient medical treatment that creates a local suction to mobilize blood flow in order to promote healing.

The physical marks on a patient's body may look like the result of domestic violence or child abuse and a physician must be thorough in ensuring that no abuse is occurring. If a physician sees these marks, he or she must make sure that no abuse is present and that the marks are indeed from these folk remedies. But they are common in Southeast Asian immigrants and usually not a sign of abuse. Answer: C

3. During a deployment, a military provider is the only physician at a forward operating base caring for approximately 500–750 military personnel. During that deployment, the provider sees a female patient who requests to initiate oral contraceptives, citing that she is presently sexually active. The patient further discloses that the individual with whom she is sexually active is her supervisor, who is also a patient of the provider. Both personnel are married and not to each other. Over the next few months the female patient discloses to the provider that the two are having difficulties in their relationship, at the same time the provider learns that the section to which both personnel are assigned is performing in a substandard fashion, which is placing other service members at risk. What action should the physician take?

A. Continue to provide medical care to both personnel.
B. Notify the commander of the inappropriate relationship.
C. Confront one or both of the patients about the relationship and its potential impact on the unit.
D. Transfer the patient to another base.
E. Transition the patient to another provider.

Patient confidentiality is an expected right of any encounter. However, this situation highlights the dilemma for the physician of protecting patient confidentiality versus the need to protect other service members of the unit who are being placed at increased risk because of the negative effects associated with the relationship. Further, this situation highlights a conflict between two professional obligations, that of the physician and the military officer. In this case, the physician may suspect that the relationship may be negatively impacting performance, but this suspicion does not provide a reason to violate the patient's confidentiality. Therefore, the physician should continue to treat both personnel and not notify the unit leadership. The provider may consider challenging the patient who has reported the ongoing relationship about the potential impact on the unit performance but should not challenge the other partner. Answer: A

4. On the first day of a medical student's first clinical rotation, an upper-level resident introduces the student to a patient using the title "Doctor." What should the student do?

A. Immediately ask the resident to explain to the patient that she is a medical student, not a doctor.
B. Say nothing; the upper-level resident will influence the student's grade.
C. When out of the patient's earshot, ask the resident to introduce her to patients as a medical student.
D. Report the resident for unprofessional behavior to the chief resident.
E. Report the resident for unprofessional behavior to the residency program director.

The student should address the situation with the resident, by pointing out that the resident should be honest with patients. Moreover, patients should not be burdened with having to overhear discussions of intra-professional matters. Answer: C

5. A bilingual male patient who is active in a violent ethnic gang enters a drug
   rehabilitation facility and begins to create separation within the community by
   speaking in his native language with other patients during group activities. The
   medical team asks the patient to refrain from such behavior in the best interest
   of the substance recovery of all the patients in the community, including him.
   The patient says that he should have the freedom to speak his native language
   with whomever he wishes and that the team is practicing undue ethnic prejudice
   against him. How should the medical team address this issue?

   A. Ask the patient to speak quietly when he speaks in his native language.
   B. Tell the patient if he does not agree with the program rules, he can leave.
   C. Ask the patient to discuss the issue with the other patients and come to an
      agreement.
   D. Assist the patient in finding a program where all the other patients speak
      his native language.
   E. Explain to the patient that the language being spoken is a clinical issue and
      that it is in the best clinical interests of all patients to speak a common
      shared language for clear communication.

   Respect for the cultural background of the patient is an important ethical
   commitment. In this situation, the bilingual patient's choices and behavior are
   undermining his clinical care and may be viewed as a clinical "sign" in relation
   to his addiction. The patient is engaging in activities that are not conducive to his
   ability to benefit from treatment and are not advancing the treatment program's
   goals for all patients, which include communication among all members of the
   group in a safe, cohesive environment. Answer A does not address the issue that
   the patient is isolating himself and others from the group as a whole. Answers B
   and D do not address the unique needs of this patient and help him understand
   why the group dynamic is in his best interest, as well as that of the entire group.
   Answer C excludes the staff from the process. Answer E involves the patient in
   the decision-making process by creating a discussion about why this request is
   being made and how his involvement will benefit himself and others. Answer: E

6. A family medicine doctor works in a small rural town. One of her patients, a 38-year-old healthy woman who comes in annually for health maintenance visits, is always friendly and conversational with the physician when they see each other around town. After a recent conversation in the grocery store, the patient invites the physician to connect on a social networking site. How should the physician handle this invitation?

   A. Accept the invitation; declining the patient as a friend will harm the patient/physician relationship.
   B. Accept the invitation; connecting on a social networking site is no different than being friendly and conversational in the grocery store.
   C. Decline the invitation; the patient is being intrusive and needs to be reminded that they are not "friends."
   D. Decline the invitation; although the invitation may be a friendly gesture, it is important to keep the relationship professional.
   E. Do not respond to the invitation and deactivate her page on the social networking site so that such invitations do not happen again in the future.

The patient-physician relationship should remain professional in nature at all times. At times, some social interactions cannot be avoided – especially for physicians who live in a small town or serve in a specific context, such as at a workplace or on a university campus. However, purposely interacting with patients on a personal social media site goes beyond incidental interaction and is outside the realm of professional contact. The patient's intent may be innocent, but gentle education to the patient at the next office visit would be appropriate and serve to preserve the patient/physician relationship. The physician could consider deactivating her account, but this action is not necessary as long as she can preserve appropriate boundaries. Answer: D

7. A pediatrician and a gerontologist together advocate for expanded coverage by governmental and commercial payers for rehabilitation services. The two physicians argue that conditions requiring rehabilitation are prevalent, severe, and highly disabling among children and elders and that these two segments of the population receive inadequate representation in society. The physicians suggest that patients at the ends of the age spectrum do not receive the insurance benefits that adults in the prime of life receive. Which of the following ethics concepts is the primary ethical rationale behind the argument advanced by this pediatrician and gerontologist?

   A. Autonomy
   B. Beneficence
   C. Justice
   D. Nonmaleficence
   E. Respect for persons

Justice refers to the equitable distribution of resources across society, and in this case, in relation to public health. The observations that conditions requiring rehabilitation disproportionately affect children and elders and yet are not insured at the same level as other illness types are especially pertinent to the justice-based argument. The pediatrician and gerontologist also mention that conditions requiring rehabilitation are severe and highly disabling. This suggests that the two physicians also may be concerned about issues related to beneficence, compassion, dignity, and nonmaleficence, but these are not the primary rationale behind the argument made. There is no specific mention of other ethical considerations such as autonomy or honesty; these concepts are meritorious but do not relate to the argument advanced by the two colleagues. Answer: C

8. A 17-year-old high school student suffers loss of consciousness while playing varsity football. He does not remember the event and had nausea and a headache for several hours afterwards, but he has felt well for several days since. His coach mandates that he get a physician evaluation before returning to play. The physician recommends that he sit out the next game to be cautious; however, the player and his father request that he get a release to play because a college recruiter is coming to the game. They feel it is their choice to assume any risk that playing involves and that the coach overstepped his role by mandating the evaluation. What should the internist do?

   A. Formally recommend that the player sit out the game and submit the evaluation to the school.
   B. Recommend that he not play but do not submit the recommendation to the school, citing patient confidentiality.
   C. Refuse to complete the evaluation and refer the player to another physician.
   D. Complete the evaluation and recommend that the choice be up to the parent.
   E. Complete the evaluation and recommend that the choice be up to the player, because he is a "mature minor."

The physician's first priority is the health and safety of the patient, consistent with the ethical principles of nonmaleficence and beneficence. Patient autonomy can be respected by referring the patient for a second opinion. However, the physician should submit the completed evaluation to the school to uphold the principles of non-deception and, more important, nonmaleficence. Answer: A

9. A 28-year-old woman is 29 weeks pregnant with a child who is known by genetic testing to have Tay-Sachs disease. She goes into preterm labor, and the baby is born with respiratory distress. The mother is adamant that she does not want mechanical ventilation for the infant because "this way his suffering can end now." The infant's respiratory status is worsening, and the infant requires mechanical ventilation. What is the next step for the ICU team?

   A. Intubate according to the "Baby Doe regulations" that guide treatment decisions in disabled children under 1 year of age.
   B. Intubate – it is in the child's best interest and that overrides the mother's decision.
   C. Intubate and immediately call the ethics committee for a full evaluation, including the possibility of extubating if warranted.
   D. Do not intubate – the mother is the decision maker about treatment in her child.
   E. Do not intubate – it would be futile given the poor prognosis of a child with Tay-Sachs.

   In this emergency situation, not acting (i.e., not intubating) results in a nonreversible outcome of patient death. A complicated case such as this requires a more thorough evaluation of the facts, which can only occur if the baby is first intubated. The Baby Doe regulations apply to decisions regarding withholding treatment in handicapped children younger than 1 year of age. However, it is not clear how these guidelines would be applied in this case given the supplied information. Ethically speaking, the answer that would best provide the patient potential benefit and prevent immediate harm with the information given would be to intubate and call for an ethics consult to evaluate how the Baby Doe regulations apply to this individual case. Answer: C

10. A military provider is assigned to complete military disability assessments. In that role, the provider evaluates a patient who was undergoing treatment for low back pain and was referred for potential medical discharge for that condition. As part of the process, the patient is referred to a VA provider who determines the level of disability for all claimed conditions. The patient is diagnosed with traumatic brain injury during the evaluation. The patient has no previous record of diagnosis or treatment for this condition. What actions should the physician take now in completing the military medical discharge evaluation?

    A. Complete the evaluation, citing the new diagnosis.
    B. Challenge the patient about the validity of the diagnoses and demand that the patient present evidence supporting the diagnoses.

C. Contact the VA physician to request information and discuss the case including diagnoses.

D. Complete the evaluation, citing only back pain and not endorsing, diagnosing, or addressing the new diagnoses.

E. Refuse to complete any evaluation.

Unlike the civilian disability system, in which evaluators are hired by the state or other organizations and the evaluation is done on their behalf, military providers are tasked with balancing the process of completing an appropriate and accurate disability examination for the Department of Defense with serving as an advocate for service members in a patient-centric process. In this case, the provider must balance the fact that a service member may have not sought care or reported these conditions due to stigma towards seeking behavioral health assistance while in the military, or on the other end of the spectrum, this service member may be attempting to defraud the government. To balance this, the physician should not "rubber-stamp" or otherwise ignore the diagnosis nor should the physician become confrontational. Rather, the physician should seek additional information to confirm the diagnoses. One mechanism would be contacting the VA provider who completed the VA exam. Answer: C

11. A 16-year-old young woman presents with her mother to an appointment with a military OB/GYN in Alaska. The mother states that her daughter needs a birth control implant. During the evaluation and consent process, the OB/GYN learns that the patient is not sexually active and does not want the procedure, but her mother states that she does want it as "protection." The provider discusses alternatives with the patient and her mother, including oral contraceptives and injectable contraceptives, but the mother is adamant that she wants the implant placed. What should the provider do?

A. The provider should decline placing the implant and reschedule an appointment with the patient alone.

B. The provider should place the birth control implant.

C. The provider should convene an emergency meeting of the hospital ethics committee.

D. The provider should report the incident to child protective services.

E. The provider should tell the 16-year-old that she has to do what her mother wants because she is the guardian.

The fact that minors have the capacity and right to make important healthcare decisions is well established in federal and state policies. Although military treatment facilities are located on federal property and the providers in those facilities are not necessarily licensed in the local state, the military has agreed to honor the local state laws when it comes to minor consent. These laws vary between states, but in Alaska, all minors are able to consent for contraceptive services. Whereas this generally leads to a situation in which a provider prescribes a contraceptive to a minor, thus upsetting the parents; the patient also has the right to refuse contraceptive treatment. Therefore, the physician in this scenario should decline placing the implant. The physician might schedule a follow-up appointment and provide the family with educational material, but the provider should honor the wishes of the young woman, who is the patient, not the mother. Answer: A

12. A Cambodian genocide survivor is referred to a psychiatrist with a diagnosis of "psychotic disorder NOS." She has had a complete and negative physical workup. Upon interview, the patient presents with symptoms of posttraumatic stress disorder and does not have symptoms consistent with a primary psychotic disorder. The woman relates that during the night, a "ghost" comes into her room and sits on her chest while she is asleep and pins her down. She feels great panic whenever this happens. The antipsychotic medication she was prescribed has not helped these symptoms. The Cambodian translator believes that this is a commonly occurring phenomenon. How should the psychiatrist approach treatment for this patient?

A. Continue the antipsychotic because the patient is still clearly psychotic.
B. Inquire about the patient's compliance, because she is still psychotic.
C. Prescribe a sleeping medication because her presentation is more likely a primary sleep problem.
D. Request information about these phenomena from someone familiar with the culture to understand the presentation better.
E. Explain through the translator that ghosts do not exist and she is simply having nightmares.

The phenomenon that the woman describes is called *khmaoch sângkât* in Khmer, which means "ghost pushing you down." It is a culturally understood paradigm of distress that occurs in Cambodians and commonly with Cambodian trauma survivors. Western doctors understand it as a form of sleep paralysis. It is not a psychotic phenomenon and does not tend to respond to antipsychotics.

Khmaoch sângkât is a culturally understood idiom of distress. Patients believe that they are literally being haunted by ghosts (often of deceased relatives). Although Western practitioners may understand this condition as a para-sleep phenomenon, success in working with patients comes from understanding their perspective and approaching them with cultural sensitivity.

This patient is not psychotic. Compliance is always important to assess, and a sleep medication may be indicated. But understanding the phenomena in the cultural context is the most important first step to treating a person with *khmaoch sângkât*. Assuming that she is psychotic without understanding the cultural context is likely to lead to misdiagnosis and incorrect and/or harmful interventions. Answer: D

13. A patient with paraplegia has spent much of the last 3 years on a specialized spinal cord unit. He has no living relatives or close friends, and he wishes to complete an advanced directive. The patient has come to regard the unit staff as his family, and he asks his long-time personal physician to serve as his health-care proxy. Which of the following is the most appropriate response to the request and its ethical justification?

A. Agree; refusing to serve as the patient's proxy would be a breach of fiduciary duty.
B. Agree; in serving as the patient's proxy, the physician honors the professional virtues of altruism and compassion.
C. Agree; the physician should serve as the patient's proxy if hospital policy allows him to do so.
D. Disagree; acting as a proxy as well as a personal physician for the patient represents a conflict of interest and a dual role.
E. Disagree; it is against the law in many states for a physician responsible for the care of a patient to also serve as a proxy decision maker.

An advanced directive is a document that describes an individual's wishes regarding future care in the event that the person loses decisional capacity. A healthcare proxy is a type of advanced directive that serves as a legal document in which a healthcare agent is named to speak for a patient regarding healthcare if a doctor determines he or she lacks the ability to make healthcare decisions.

In general, naming a healthcare provider who is directly providing care for a patient as a healthcare proxy is strongly discouraged because it results in a dual role and is inherently a conflict of interest. A conflict of interest in medicine is a situation in which a physician has competing roles, relationships, or interests that could potentially interfere with the ability to care for patients. It is crucial for medical professionals to recognize and respond to these conflicts ethically. In this scenario, the physician would potentially be at odds with his fiduciary duty towards his patient and his role as a possible benefactor from his patient, if the patient were to lose his decisional capacity.

Nonetheless, although state laws vary, it is generally mandated that a physician can serve as a healthcare proxy as long as he or she is named before the patient is admitted into the hospital where the physician is employed. After the patient is admitted to the hospital, the patient may only legally name as a healthcare proxy a healthcare worker who is an employee of that hospital if the worker is a direct relative of the patient. Finally, if a physician does indeed become the healthcare proxy, the physician cannot be the person to determine the patient's decisional capacity. These safeguards are designed to limit the potential ethical dilemmas rising from this dual role and conflict of interest. Answer: D

14. A surgeon evaluated a patient for a major procedure. The patient appeared to be mildly confused; however, he did not show signs of objection when the doctor proposed the operation. The patient then signed the consent form, and most of the patient's family members were present at the time. The doctor would like to schedule the operation. Which issue may be especially problematic in this scenario?

   A. The patient may not have adequate decisional capacity to consent to the risks and benefits of the procedure because of his confusion.
   B. The surgeon should have waited to discuss the operation because not all family members were present at the time the patient signed the consent form.
   C. The surgeon placed his need for scheduling convenience ahead of the patient's needs.
   D. None; the patient signed a consent form, so it is assumed that he did not have any objections to the procedure.
   E. None; the patient needed the surgery for his condition immediately and to delay the operation would be unethical.

Informed consent for any medical or surgical intervention encompasses three major categories: (1) information sharing, (2) decisional capacity, and (3) voluntarism. All of these elements should be addressed during the informed consent discussion. Because the patient shows symptoms of confusion, the surgeon should use careful clinical judgment to explore further both the cause and the extent of this patient's potential cognitive and other impairments. For instance, the patient could have various medical comorbidities that are temporarily affecting his mental status, such as the acute onset of delirium. Likewise, the patient could have an undiagnosed mental illness or could be developing dementia. Further assessment should be conducted to evaluate the patient's ability to consent to the procedure.

Additionally, the standard for informed consent depends on the nature of the decision to be made. Higher risk decisions necessitate stricter, more rigorous standards. Because a major operation poses significant risks to the patient, the "sliding scale" approach to informed consent should warrant a higher stringency of consent standards. Answer: A

15. An attending physician has just discharged from the emergency room an adolescent girl who wrote an essay in which she discussed a shooting at a school. He does not believe that the patient is a threat to anyone, and the patient has no specific plans to commit any violent acts at her school. A consulting psychiatrist concurs with his conclusion. Later that evening, the attending physician receives a call from a senior professor of medicine who is married to the principal of the high school. The professor asks the attending physician to tell him about the case, specifically whether or not the patient has access to a weapon. How should the attending physician handle this call?

A. Tell the professor that he understands his concern but has an obligation to maintain the privacy of his patients and is unable to discuss the case.
B. Tell the professor that the student does not have access to a weapon.
C. Tell the professor that the principal can talk to the student at school if she is concerned.
D. Tell the professor that the girl only wrote an essay, and there is no need to worry.
E. Report the behavior of the professor to the dean of the medical school.

This case highlights the importance of patient privacy and confidential information that may be shared in a clinical setting. The professor appears concerned about the safety of others, who may be at risk because of information that the patient has shared. Patients should be informed that all information is kept confidential, unless there is a risk of danger to the patient or other people. In this case, the attending physician and the consulting psychiatrist have determined that there is no risk of danger, and on the basis of the clinical information, the patient is safe to leave the hospital without the physicians alerting the authorities about what she has shared. Sharing this information with another provider who is not caring for this patient, even if that provider practices in the same medical center, would be unethical and break the obligation of privacy to this patient. Shifting the burden to the school is also incorrect. The provider's duty was to evaluate the girl's psychiatric state in the emergency room, and involving others such as her school authorities in the situation is beyond that scope. Answer: A

16. A hospitalist admits a 78-year-old Japanese woman with abdominal pain and weight loss. The medical workup reveals advanced stomach cancer. The woman has decision-making capacity but defers to her son as the head of the family. The woman's son requests that the internist does not disclose to the patient that she has cancer but instead tell her she has an ulcer that can be treated with medications and diet change. Which of the following is the most appropriate response to the request and its ethical justification?

    A. Agree; the son as the head of the family has the legal right to make decisions on his mother's behalf and may determine what medical information is disclosed or withheld.
    B. Agree; the mother has indicated that her son is the head of the family and has implicitly deferred medical decisions to him as her surrogate decision maker.
    C. Disagree; the internist must first speak to the woman and her son together and ensure she wishes the son and not another family member to serve as her surrogate.
    D. Disagree; the internist must first speak to the woman alone and ask her if she wishes to be informed of her medical condition or to have the information be communicated to her son.
    E. Disagree; the patient has decision-making capacity, and the internist has the ethical obligation to disclose the patient's diagnosis so that the patient can make informed decisions regarding her treatment. The son has no legal standing or ethical warrant to request his mother not to be told the truth.

Professional standards of medical practice are often based on Western cultural norms and may come into conflict within the practice of cross-cultural medicine. In this scenario, the clinician should identify the conflict between the ethical principles of respecting patient autonomy and veracity. Because the patient is deemed to have full decisional capacity, she is an autonomous patient; that is, she has the ability to make deliberated or reasoned decisions and she can act on the basis of those decisions. Veracity refers to honesty, or conveying information and meaning truthfully, without misrepresentation through deceit, bias, or omission.

The internist must take into consideration different cultural interpretations of autonomy. For instance, it is not uncommon for patients of Japanese descent to enable family members to make medical decisions for them from the belief that their families know what is best for them. Patients will even sometimes expect family members to withhold the direct disclosure of a terminal illness diagnosis to protect them from emotional harm. Thus, in order to ensure that the patient's wishes are truly respected in this scenario, the internist appropriately verifies these wishes directly with the patient. Patient preferences should always be viewed and interpreted within a clinical framework, the patient's choices should be explored, and culturally sensitive interventions should be considered.

In this scenario, if the patient tells the internist that she will continue to defer all medical information and decisions to her son, it would be appropriate for the physician to discuss alternative ways of approaching the patient that would not eventually harm her. For instance, it is illegal to distribute medications with no indication, as the son is proposing the internist to do, and the patient's trust in both the medical community and her son could potentially be compromised. Answer: D

17. A 47-year-old patient who is awaiting a renal transplant is admitted to the intensive care unit in complete heart block and acute-on-chronic renal failure. She is alert and oriented, appropriately conversational, without a known psychiatric history. She refuses urgent placement of a pacemaker for her heart block because she believes "the real problem is my kidneys." She has no healthcare power of attorney named, and despite several attempts to educate her on the life-saving indication for a pacemaker, she repeatedly states, "I do not want to talk about this now. I am not ready. Things will be fine." What is the next step for the ICU team?

    A. Give the patient time to think about her choice.
    B. Contact hospital administration to help determine who should be making decisions on behalf of the patient because she does not have a healthcare power of attorney.
    C. Ask the patient to elect a healthcare power of attorney.
    D. Call for an ethics consult to decide who should be making medical decisions for the patient.
    E. Evaluate the patient's capacity to refuse a pacemaker or call a consultant to perform the evaluation.

There is reason to question the patient's capacity given her refusal to engage with the treatment team for the care of her urgent medical issue. Although this situation itself does not indicate that she lacks capacity, further evaluation is warranted. Given that the medical situation is urgent, allowing the patient more time would be irresponsible without knowing if she actually has capacity to make this decision, which is consistent with the ethical principle of nonmaleficence. Before assigning a healthcare power of attorney or calling an ethics committee or hospital administration to determine a surrogate decision maker, the ICU staff should respect the patient's autonomy by first determining if she does in fact lack capacity through a thorough evaluation. Answer: E

18. A patient develops vision loss after an eye surgery, and the ophthalmologist tells the patient that the vision loss must be vascular in nature because there were no ocular complications in surgery. The vascular surgeon finds that the minimal level of vascular pathology cannot account for the level of vision loss and suspects that the ophthalmologist who performed the original operation may not have been truthful with the patient about complications. The patient is desperate to recover his sight and wants the vascular surgeon to repair his minor pathology despite the vascular surgeon's warnings that the repair will likely not improve his vision. What should the vascular surgeon do?

A. Tell the patient that there must have been a mistake during his eye surgery and refer him back to the ophthalmologist.
B. Discuss the case with the ophthalmologist and determine the best course of care for the patient, addressing all possible scenarios.
C. Perform the vascular surgery because the patient deserves to have the care he requests.
D. Refuse to perform vascular surgery and refer the patient to an optometrist for glasses.
E. Perform the vascular surgery under the condition that the patient agrees to not hold the vascular surgeon responsible for any complications.

This scenario presents the question of how to maneuver between a patient's best interest and the professional responsibility between medical colleagues. When another clinician's advice or judgment is thought to be potentially inaccurate, it is best to keep open communication between all parties involved. Option A assumes that the vascular surgeon knows what happened during the ocular surgery, which is incorrect, and shifts blame where there is still an unknown. Option C puts the patient at risk for unnecessary harm. The physician's responsibility is to choose treatment options on the basis of his or her judgment, not solely on patient preference or request. Option D avoids the conflict and does not address the patient's request for surgery or the possibility that the previous surgery had done harm. Option B is the best choice, because it allows each physician to discuss the case on the basis of his or her area of expertise and provides an open discussion of possibilities. Answer: B

19. A gynecologist assesses a non-English-speaking Bosnian concentration camp survivor for her chronic pelvic pain. The translator is a Serbian woman. The patient is uncooperative with the interview and clearly emotionally distressed. She does not endorse any symptoms during the interview. What is a likely explanation for the patient's poor engagement?

    A. The patient is no longer experiencing symptoms.
    B. The patient is malingering.
    C. The patient is not comfortable with the translator because of cultural and political differences.
    D. The patient is not comfortable with the gynecologist.
    E. The patient has a personality disorder.

    Often in cross-cultural medicine, translation services are limited. It is important to consider the relationship between the patient and the translator, because issues between them may limit the patient's willingness to disclose information. A common language does not always suggest a common religious, ethnic, or cultural background. In this scenario, many Bosnian clients will be cautious or unwilling to disclose personal information with a Serbian translator, even though both speak Serbo-Croatian, because of the history of conflict in the former Yugoslavia. Answer: C

20. A 29-year-old HIV-positive woman who has lived with the virus for 15 years has developed severe lipodystrophy, a deforming condition characterized by the wasting of subcutaneous fat in the face and extremities and visceral fat accumulation in the abdomen. She is reclusive and on permanent disability due to other HIV-related conditions. She denies anhedonia and continues to enjoy knitting and playing with her two cats. She takes her medications, eats well, and manages her activities of daily living. She reports her mood as "good." She has intermittent diarrhea with rare episodes of incontinence, fatigue, pain due to neuropathy, and avascular necrosis. Her pain is now under good control, but she remains limited in her ability to ambulate. Her conditions are chronic. She is cognitively intact and capable of making healthcare decisions. She confides in her physician that she has decided to stop taking her HIV medications. She understands that she may very well die within a few years if she stops her medications, but she reports, "This life is not what I had expected. I am ready to move on. I am at peace with this decision." What might her physician do?

A. Place her on an involuntary psychiatric hold. She has expressed suicidal ideation with a plan to end her life.
B. Place her on an involuntary psychiatric hold. She is gravely disabled, lacks good judgment, and is unable to make rational decisions about her medical care.
C. Continue to prescribe the recommended treatment for her, because discontinuing the HIV medications would constitute physician-assisted suicide.
D. Discontinue the HIV medications and her pain medications. Because she is terminating the HIV medications, the physician no longer has the duty to treat her pain.
E. Discontinue the HIV medications and provide symptomatic relief as she becomes increasingly ill.

This patient is offering clear evidence of informed refusal of care. Given that this patient is decisionally capable, the physician must abide by her wishes. Informed refusal of care differs for physician-assisted suicide and euthanasia. Physician-assisted suicide is a concept in which the physician provides a patient with a substance at a lethal amount for her to take on her own. Physician-assisted suicide is not euthanasia, in which the physician directly and with compassionate intent acts to end the life of a person with an incurable and progressive disease that will cause imminent death.

Evaluating the woman's decisional capacity is an important consideration in this scenario. One must take into account the chronic conditions that can affect the brain such as HIV encephalopathy and primary CNS lymphoma. But if the woman shows no signs or symptoms suggesting that these pathologies are present, she has decisional capacity, and her choice must be respected. The physician should then focus the discussion primarily on issues pertaining to her future palliative care management.

In accordance with the philosophy of palliative care, it is vital to address all of the woman's physical, psychological, and spiritual concerns, as well as those of her family members and friends who share a close connection with her. Any cultural issues surrounding end-of-life care should also be respected. Additionally, advanced directive planning should be discussed and documented, ensuring that her wishes are upheld as her disease progresses. The woman should understand the consequences of her decision to forgo medical therapy, such as the opportunistic infections that will eventually overwhelm her immune system as her CD4 counts drop. Finally, a hospice consultation may be helpful, especially if it is determined that without her HIV medications, she likely has fewer than 6 months to live. Answer: E

21. An Iraqi refugee presented to his primary care physician with a prior diagnosis of type 2 diabetes. The patient's blood glucose levels are poorly controlled despite treatment with oral hypoglycemic. The Arabic translator and case manager report that she believes the client has not been taking the medication as prescribed. What approach should the physician use to improve the treatment plan?

    A. Change medications because the patient does not like the treatment plan.
    B. Confront the patient and insist on compliance.
    C. Find out why the patient is not taking the medication.
    D. Recommend a traditional healer.
    E. Refuse to treat the patient because of the liability issues with non-compliance.

Compliance with medication is a major issue in cross-cultural medicine. Medication checks can be very challenging for physicians because of reports of good compliance in the context of poor compliance. It is important for the physician to understand the patient's perception of the medication's role in the treatment and to invite very open communication about the expectations of medications' efficacy and side effects. Answer: C

22. A reserve physician works at a military medical facility for his activated time. When he is not an activated reserve officer, the physician works at a civilian dual-diagnosis residential substance abuse clinic. During an appointment with the reserve physician, a military service member endorses anxiety symptoms and ongoing struggles with alcohol abuse. What would be the appropriate action for the physician to take?

    A. Report the substance abuse to the commanding officer.
    B. Refer the service member to the local military alcohol and substance abuse program.
    C. Arrange for the service member to receive treatment at the civilian dual-diagnosis residential substance abuse clinic where the physician works.
    D. Ignore the alcohol abuse claim and keep it out of the medical record.
    E. Treat the anxiety without addressing the substance abuse issue.

Reserve providers who also have positions that interact with or are part of the federal government must be cognizant of the potential conflict of interest that their various roles might create. In this scenario, the physician should address the substance abuse issue, and not expect it to be identified by the next provider, but what might seem like an "extra effort" for caring for the service member by coordinating with a specific program might undermine the referral process and create a potential financial benefit to the physician. Thus, the physician should refer the service member to substance abuse treatment, either locally or to a residential program, depending on the severity of the symptoms, but not to a specific program. Answer: B

23. A 20-year-old Asian female with developmental delay and cerebral palsy is admitted to the hospital following a generalized tonic-clonic seizure. She is diagnosed with epilepsy by a neurologist. Her mother, who cares for her and is her legal guardian, wants to take her home to be treated traditionally. When asked if her daughter has had seizures before, the mother responds that she experienced a similar episode two other times in the last year, but the mother did not seek medical assistance. The mother tells the neurologist that her daughter's seizures result from "sadness" because she is not married and has no children. The mother plans to find the daughter a husband to relieve her "sadness," which will eradicate her seizures. There is no evidence that the mother has abused or neglected her daughter. What should the neurologist do?

A. Let the mother take her daughter home because she is her legal guardian.
B. Ask the daughter if she wants to find a husband.
C. Educate the mother about her daughter's diagnosis and explain how her daughter may benefit from treatment.
D. Tell the mother that you disagree and will not discharge her daughter.
E. Ask the mother about her negative experiences with Western medicine.

In this scenario, the patient's mother provides for her because of her developmental delay and is also making the decisions about her treatment for her new diagnosis of epilepsy. However, the neurologist's obligation is to provide the best care possible for this patient, and letting her mother dismiss medical treatment would be negligent. Option B is impractical because the patient currently cannot care for herself and her opinion about marriage is irrelevant to her medical care. Discussing previous experiences with the mother is also not relevant and might create more negativity between the mother and the provider. Option C allows the mother to become part of the treatment process and involves her in the care of the patient, which will provide the best long-term outcomes for the patient, because her mother will better understand the recommendations being made. Answer: C

24. A female medical student enters a patient's room to take a history and perform a physical examination. As soon as she comes through the door, the patient says that his bladder is "full to burstin'." He then adds that, as a nurse, she needs to get him the bedpan quickly. How should the student respond?

A. Take offense at the patient's sexism and get the nurse.
B. Promptly get him the bedpan and assist him to urinate as necessary.
C. Press the call button for the nurse to come.
D. State that she is there to take a history and perform a physical.
E. State that she is a medical student and that his request is for nursing help.

The professional virtue of self-effacement requires the student to ignore the fact she has been assumed to be a nurse. The student has a fiduciary obligation to provide the patient immediate assistance. Answer: B

25. A researcher recruits patients for a clinical trial. A severely ill patient volunteers for the trial, saying, "This treatment has to help me get better." With what misconception is the patient's statement most consistent?

A. All volunteers are allowed to participate in research.
B. Medical research is a purely altruistic activity.
C. Researchers pressure potential participants to enroll.
D. Research volunteers are certain to receive better treatments than are clinically available.
E. Research protocols fully safeguard participants.

A common misconception concerning medical research is that clinical protocols are certain to provide research participants with direct therapeutic benefits. In reality, investigational therapies often fail to show significant advantages over standard treatments. Moreover, to be ethical, under most circumstances studies are structured to answer the unresolved question of whether or not a particular intervention is helpful – that is, the condition of "equipoise" is necessary for an ethically sound scientific design.

The overestimation of the benefits of research participation has been termed the "therapeutic misconception." In both psychiatric and nonpsychiatric research participants, the therapeutic misconception leads to inappropriate expectations regarding the degree of individualization of the treatment and the nature or likelihood of therapeutic benefit. Research participants demonstrating this misconception may be unrealistically optimistic about the benefits of the experimental intervention. Often, these individuals also minimize the risks associated with the experimental agent. Investigators themselves may be influenced by the fallacy as they recruit participants or enroll them in specific arms of a trial.

To minimize the impact of the therapeutic misconception, researchers must use the informed consent process to educate potential participants about the goals of the trial (i.e., to seek to answer a scientific question) and how they differ from the goals of clinical care (i.e., to seek to benefit the individual patient). Potential participants must be thoroughly informed about the elements of the research protocol that involve risks and about nonroutine procedures and should be carefully educated about the concepts of randomization and blinding, if applicable. Answer: D

26. A faculty member in a pediatrics department primarily works in a general outpatient clinic but rotates on the inpatient service for 2 weeks at the local children's hospital. One of the faculty member's patients is a 16-year-old girl with cystic fibrosis. The pediatric pulmonology fellow tells the faculty member that he is concerned about the patient because she is not cooperating with her inpatient medical treatment plan and has a long history of nonadherence with her treatment. When the faculty member interviews the patient, she complains that she does not like the fellow because he has a poor bedside manner and has not given her a proper explanation about her treatment plan. Later, the faculty member overhears two nurses complaining about the pulmonology fellow and his inability to communicate in a respectful manner. How should the faculty member handle this situation?

A. Suggest to the family of the patient that they find a new pulmonologist.
B. Explain to the pulmonologist that the patient may adhere better to the treatment if he had a better bedside manner.
C. Provide the patient with an explanation about her pulmonary treatment.
D. Ask the nurses to give examples of the pulmonologist's inability to communicate.
E. Educate the pulmonologist about communicating difficult medical information to children in a developmentally and emotionally appropriate manner, framed as recommendations from a consultant who specializes in this area.

In this scenario, the faculty member confronts the challenge of an early-career colleague who may not be fully informed about working with children who have serious medical illness in a manner that addresses their emotional and mental needs. Involving other staff in the discussion (Option D) would be inappropriate because the important clinical information came from the patient, who not only wants an explanation of her current treatment (Option C) but also wants to change the pattern developed between her and the pulmonology fellow. Suggesting that the patient change pulmonologists (Option A) could occur later if the situation cannot be resolved but does not address the present question from the provider or the concerns of the patient. Option B does not educate the pulmonology fellow about how to better communicate with this patient. Option E allows for the pulmonology fellow to improve communication with the patient, enables the patient to feel that her needs were heard by the faculty member and are being met by the pulmonologist, and establishes patterns of communication that can be used in the future. Answer: E

27. A psychiatrist provides medication management in an outpatient clinic at an academic medical center. She treats a patient who receives individual therapy with a psychologist who is a professor in the department. The patient routinely requests medication changes from the psychiatrist. The psychiatrist learns that the patient often discusses medication issues with the psychologist during their therapy sessions. According to the patient, the psychologist has been making these suggestions regarding medication adjustments. Which of the following is the most appropriate course of action for the psychiatrist?

   A. Complain to the department chairman about the psychologist's unprofessional behavior.
   B. Say that she can no longer treat the patient if the patient continues to discuss medication issues with the psychologist.
   C. Complain about the professor's behavior to the state licensing board for psychologists.
   D. Warn her colleagues not to refer patients to this psychologist, who clearly has boundary issues.
   E. Call the psychologist to discuss what transpired in the visit with the patient.

   In healthcare systems where several providers may be involved in the care of a patient, opportunities for miscommunication and confusion are rife. Before the psychiatrist assumes that the psychologist is indeed directing the patient's requests for medication changes and acting outside his scope of practice, the psychiatrist needs to communicate directly with the psychologist about the patient's disclosure. Answer: E

28. A medical student serves as a research assistant and mentee for a senior faculty member and receives minimum wage payment for gathering data and data analysis. The student develops a novel project with her mentor, gathers the data, analyzes the data, and then prepares a manuscript, which the senior faculty member submits to a journal as a sole-authored paper, not including the student as author or coauthor. The student confronts the senior faculty member, who responds: "This project was my idea and I got the funding for it. You were a paid research assistant. Your paycheck was your reward, not the manuscript." On what grounds should the student have received credit as a coauthor?

   A. Because she was paid to participate in the project.
   B. Because she helped conceptualize the project, gather and analyze the data, and write up the project.
   C. Because she is a medical student.
   D. Because she is the mentee of the senior faculty member.
   E. Because she gathered the data.

This student helped develop the project, gather and analyze the data, and develop the manuscript. According to authorship guidelines, the student qualifies as a coauthor because of her participation in each of these steps. The fact that she receives a paycheck for work at minimum wage is not relevant to the authorship determination. Answer: B

29. A resident physician in a teaching hospital frequently drinks socially. He admits to drinking to blackout regularly but rationalizes that it "never affects my work." He comes to work with a black eye after a night out drinking with friends that ended in a physical altercation. Another resident expresses concern to him about his drinking, and he becomes defensive, citing his friends' view of his drinking as "normal." What is the most appropriate action for the coresident to take?

A. Discuss the situation with a senior faculty member whose specialty is substance abuse to determine the likelihood that the resident's drinking meets criteria for abuse or dependence.
B. Confront him about his drinking in front of his peers because he responded with denial when approached one-on-one.
C. Inform the hospital's physician well-being committee because it investigates possible impairment of medical staff and trainees.
D. Leave an anonymous note for the residency training program director that alcoholism is a problem among the staff members.
E. Report the resident's behavior to the state medical board.

In this scenario, the resident's drinking is clearly concerning and may be affecting his personal life, health, and work, but there is no clear evidence of occupational impairment with patient safety in jeopardy or ethical breeches. Alcohol-related incidents of blackouts and physical altercation, however, usually indicate a level of intake that very likely has led, or will lead at some point in the future, to professional impairment. A hospital's physician well-being committee may be the best body to investigate possible impairment and follow through with appropriate referrals and monitoring, ideally taking a supportive, remediation-centered approach, rather than a punitive one. Answer: C

30. A family physician in an urban private practice treats a 20-year-old woman whose primary complaint is a progressively worsening feeling of depression over the past several months. She works for the local ballet company and cites both job dissatisfaction and a low sense of self-worth as the main contributors to her depression. The physician serves as a member of the board for the ballet company. What should the physician do?

    A. Begin treatment with a medication without mentioning the role on the board, because this role is not a conflict of interest.
    B. Refer the patient to another primary care provider or a psychiatrist for treatment because of this conflict of interest.
    C. Tell the patient about the role on the board and enable her to decide if she feels comfortable continuing treatment.
    D. Treat the patient after resigning from the board.
    E. Provide medication management for the patient but refer her to a therapist for psychotherapy.

    Full disclosure of the physician's involvement on the board is warranted to value the patient's autonomy in choosing a treatment provider. Not disclosing this role could be viewed as a form of deception and may harm the patient-physician relationship if the role is discovered. Being on the board of something like a ballet company is not itself a conflict of interest for the physician as long as the board does not directly make contract decisions or supervise the individual in treatment. There is no indication for the patient to take a leave of absence in this scenario, and a contingent agreement for treatment compromises patient autonomy. Answer: C

31. A 58-year-old man with newly diagnosed pancreatic cancer begins treatment with an oncologist. During the interview the oncologist learns that the patient is a relatively well-known businessman who has been in the news lately for a personal scandal. The oncologist is curious to know more about the scandal and considers searching the Internet for information. Is this search ethical?

    A. No; it is never relevant or ethical to look up a patient on the Internet because it is a breach of trust.
    B. No; this information is irrelevant to the man's healthcare.
    C. Yes, if the patient signed a general release of information.
    D. Yes; information on the Internet is public domain and therefore ethical for anyone to view.
    E. Yes, as long as the information does not change the care the patient receives.

    The ethical principles of beneficence and nonmaleficence are the focus in this scenario. Although the information is in the public domain, the oncologist's intent in looking it up is not to benefit to the patient and could in fact harm the patient-physician relationship. Answer: B

32. An English-speaking Salvadorian woman who survived a gang rape is over-whelmed by shame in the idea that she is guilty of "sin" and therefore "unclean before God" because of the sexual implications of her trauma. She tells her psychiatrist that only God can forgive her, but she believes that God will not do so. She wants to go to a priest in addition to the psychiatrist because she believes that only a priest can absolve her. How should the psychiatrist respond to the woman?

A. The psychiatrist should deemphasize the religious beliefs since they are harmful to her psychological state.
B. The psychiatrist should tell the woman not to go to a priest.
C. The psychiatrist should explore with the woman her guilt around the sexual violence, incorporating the woman's religious beliefs to maximize the therapeutic process.
D. The psychiatrist should refer her to a Spanish-speaking psychiatrist.
E. The psychiatrist should focus only on management with antidepressants.

Some problems may present as mental health in the eyes of an American-trained psychiatrist but be experienced otherwise by the patient, such as when a patient attaches religious or spiritual meaning to an event. From a patient's perspective, the spiritual issue may have no place in a psychiatric treatment plan. The woman in the scenario may find more relief from a blessing or reassurance from a priest than from her psychiatrist. Still, the psychiatrist can process the themes in therapy. Some cross-cultural mental health programs collaborate with religious leaders around interventions for patients who have experienced trauma. Answer: C

33. A child psychiatrist works closely with a 14-year-old girl from Iran who has metastatic Ewing's disease and is unlikely to live more than another 2 to 3 weeks. Her parents tell the treatment team that they do not want their daughter to know about her diagnosis or prognosis. They add that in their culture, children are protected from medical information and that parents make all of the medical decisions. The patient has been having panic attacks. She tells the psychiatrist that she does not know what is wrong with her but is afraid that she might die. She also tells the psychiatrist that if she were going to die, she would like to know so that she can say goodbye to her friends. How should the psychiatrist respond?

A. Tell the parents that the treatment team is obligated to tell the patient that she has 2–3 weeks to live.
B. With the parents, develop a plan that reveals enough information to the patient to help her understand her situation and also reflects the parents' concerns and cultural needs.
C. Tell the patient to say goodbye to her friends but do not give her any additional information.
D. Ask the parents to tell the patient about her diagnosis.
E. Agree with the parents that the patient should not be told any information about her diagnosis.

This scenario illustrates the conflict that may arise when parents wish to withhold information that their child may want to know. Here, the patient is suffering from panic attacks because of the withheld information. Option E would likely leave the patient with ongoing anxiety. Options A and D disregard the parents' needs and their involvement in their child's care. Option C would likely instill a significant amount of fear in the patient. By choosing option B, the psychiatrist can work with the family and the patient to develop a plan that will be best overall. Answer: B

34. A commander asks a military unit medical provider to supply a list of all soldiers who are diagnosed with obstructive sleep apnea. The commander notes the deployment limitations for soldiers with obstructive sleep apnea and is concerned about the impact on unit readiness and strength. What actions should the medical provider take?

   A. Tell the commander that she cannot provide any information.
   B. Tell the commander that she is unable to evaluate sleep apnea in her patients.
   C. Give the commander a list of soldiers who have deployment-limiting conditions.
   D. Give the commander a list of soldiers with obstructive sleep apnea.
   E. Give the commander access to the medical records of the patients with sleep apnea.

Medical providers must be cautious in releasing medical information, especially without patients' written consent. The Health Insurance Portability and Accountability Act (HIPAA) has a military exception, however, which allows commanders to be aware of duty limitations or conditions that impact military service members' ability to perform their duty. In general, that release is limited to a diagnosis, prognosis, and duty limitations. Therefore, the provider should either give an aggregate response so that the unit commander has an understanding of the scope of the issue or provide a list of those who have deployment limitations, because this information affects unit readiness and is covered under the HIPAA exception. Answer: C

35. A resident has conducted diabetes research with a highly regarded senior researcher who has been a good mentor and made key contributions to a research manuscript she is preparing. He requests that she involves an assistant professor on the paper as a coauthor. The manuscript is almost ready for submission to a peer-reviewed journal. She learns from another colleague that this assistant professor is coming up for promotion and "needs more publications on her CV." The resident thinks that the assistant professor's input at this stage would be minimal and not meet criteria for authorship. Which of the following is the most appropriate course of action for the resident?

   A. Ignore the request and submit the manuscript.
   B. Discuss the rationale behind the request and, if necessary, raise concerns regarding adding another author at this stage of preparation.
   C. Invite the assistant professor as a coauthor.
   D. Notify the assist ant professor that the paper does not need her input.
   E. Complain to the department chair about the mentor's request.

Authorship on scientific manuscripts is a contentious issue. Fortunately, clear guidelines on what constitutes authorship on a manuscript are now available. Authorship credit should be based on (1) substantial contributions to conception and design, acquisition of data, or analysis and interpretation of data; (2) drafting the paper or revising it critically for important intellectual content; and (3) final approval of the version to be published. Authors should meet conditions 1, 2, and 3. Although the assistant professor does not appear to meet criteria for authorship, the resident should seek more information from her mentor about the reason for the request. Answer: B

Recommended Reading

American Medical Association Council on Ethical and Judicial Affairs: Code of Medical Ethics: Current Opinions with Annotations, 2010–2011 edition. Chicago: American Medical Association; 2010.

Aroche J, Coello M. Ethnocultural considerations in the treatment of refugees. In: Wilson JP, Drozdek B, editors. Broken spirits: The treatment of traumatized asylum seekers, refugees, war and torture victims. New York: Brunner-Routledge; 2004. p. 53–81.

Beauchamp TL, Childress JF. Principles of biomedical ethics. 6th ed. New York: Oxford University Press; 2008.

Boyd KM, Higgs R, Pinching AJ. The new dictionary of medical ethics. London: BMJ Publishing; 1997.

Brems C, Johnson ME, Warner TD, Roberts LW. Patient requests and provider suggestions for alternative treatments as reported by rural and urban care providers. Complement Ther Med. 2006;14:10–19.

Furrow BR, Greaney TL, Johnson SH, Jost TS, Schwartz RL. Bioethics: Health care law and ethics. 6th ed. St. Paul: Thomson West; 2008.

Grisso T, Appelbaum P. Assessing competence to consent to treatment: A guide for physicians and other health professionals. New York: Oxford University Press; 1998.

Hoop JG, DiPasquale T, Hernandez J, Roberts LW. Ethics and culture in mental health care. Ethics and Behav. 2008;18(4):353–72.

Hoop J, Roberts LW, Green Hammond K. Genetic testing of stored biological samples: views of 570 U.S. workers. Genet Test Mol Biomarkers. 2009;13(3):331–7.

Jonsen AR, Siegler M, Winslade WJ. Clinical ethics: A practical approach to ethical decisions in clinical medicine. 7th ed. New York: McGraw-Hill; 2010.

Koenig HG. Spirituality in patient care. 2nd ed. Philadelphia: Templeton Foundation Press; 2007.

Kushe H, Singer P. A companion to bioethics. Oxford: Blackwell; 1998.

Kushner TK, Thomasma DC. Ward ethics dilemmas for medical students and doctors in training. Cambridge: Cambridge University Press; 2001.

Lo B. Resolving ethical dilemmas, a guide for clinicians. 3rd ed. Philadelphia: Lippincott Williams & Wilkins; 2005.

Mappes TA, Zembaty JS, editors. Biomedical ethics. 2nd ed. New York: McGraw-Hill; 1986.

Pierce J, Randels G. Contemporary bioethics: A reader with cases. Oxford: Oxford University Press; 2010.

Roberts LW, Dyer A. A concise guide to ethics in mental health care. Washington, DC: American Psychiatric Publishing; 2004.

Roberts LW, Dunn LB. Ethical considerations in caring for women with substance use disorders. Obstet Gynecol Clin North Am. 2003;30(3):559–82.

Roberts LW, Fromm LM. Physicians and sexuality. In: Mattox JH, editor. Core textbook of obstetrics and gynecology. 10th ed. St. Louis: Mosby Yearbook Press; 1998. p. 502–507.

Sperry L. Dictionary of ethical and legal terms and issues: The essential guide for mental health professionals. London: Routledge; 2007.

Tseng W, Streltzer J, editors. Cultural competence in clinical psychiatry. Washington, DC: American Psychiatric Publishing; 2004.

Veatch RM. The basics of bioethics. 2nd ed. Upper Saddle River: Prentice Hall; 2003.

Chapter 7
Questions on Core Concepts

Laura Weiss Roberts and Daryn Reicherter

This chapter contains questions from across medical disciplines. The questions are designed to test the learner's understanding of the core concepts of professionalism and ethics in medicine. Correct answers are listed at the end of the section. The learner may refer back to the relevant chapter in Part I for the conceptual framework.

1. A woman who practices the Jehovah's Witness religion has a clear wish not to receive blood products, even under life-threatening conditions. She has stated this wish verbally and also signed a written statement with the same wish. She is pregnant. Eight hours after being admitted to the labor and delivery service, she is taken to the operating room for a seemingly uncomplicated Cesarean section. The surgeons encounter more blood loss than they had anticipated and decide that the patient needs a hysterectomy. The patient is put under general anesthesia and a stat hemoglobin is sent. The patient's hemoglobin is 5, and more blood loss is anticipated. The surgeons would like to give the patient a blood transfusion, but the patient is unable to communicate. What is the most appropriate action?

Contributing authors: Laura Weiss Roberts, M.D., M.A., Daryn Reicherter, M.D., Victor G. Carrion, M.D., Jodi K. Casados, M.D., John H. Coverdale, M.D., M.Ed., Michelle Goldsmith, M.D., M.A., Joseph B. Layde, M.D., J.D., Sermsak Lolak, M.D., Lawrence McCullough, Ph.D., Lawrence M. McGlynn, M.D., Christine Moutier, M.D., Mark T. Wright, M.D.

L.W. Roberts, M.D., M.A. (✉) • D. Reicherter, M.D.
Department of Psychiatry and Behavioral Sciences,
Stanford University School of Medicine, Stanford, CA, USA
e-mail: RobertsL@stanford.edu

© Springer Science+Business Media New York 2015   113
L.W. Roberts, D. Reicherter (eds.), *Professionalism and Ethics in Medicine*,
DOI 10.1007/978-1-4939-1686-3_7

A. Move forward with the blood transfusion because it may be lifesaving, and the patient clearly must not have understood the ramifications of her decision at an earlier time when she was not facing a life-threatening emergency.

B. Consult with the patient's family members to verify that her wish to decline all blood products is consistent with her religious beliefs and agreeable to the family.

C. Obtain a biomedical ethics consult, because the physician must "do no harm" and, by withholding blood transfusion, may harm the patient.

D. Proceed with all efforts to prevent blood loss, including possible hysterectomy, without providing blood transfusion, because the patient has clearly stated her wishes.

E. Consult with the patient's next of kin in order to obtain revised consent.

2–3.   For each of the following scenarios, indicate whether or not the physician's conduct is considered ethically acceptable in light of the recommendations of the American Medical Association Council on Ethical and Judicial Affairs.

A. Acceptable
B. Not Acceptable

2.   ____ A resident begins a dating relationship with a recently referred patient in her clinic.

3.   ____ A late-career physician begins a dating relationship with a patient.

4.   The neighbor of an emergency medicine physician shares that he and his wife have hired a new au pair, who will be living in their house. The physician realizes that he has seen the au pair in his emergency room several times. She has come in with different complaints but consistently has been intoxicated with alcohol and has a history of accidents and self-harm. What should the physician do?

A. The physician should tell his patient that she may see him in the neighborhood, because they will be living near each other.

B. The physician should review the circumstance with a trusted mentor or supervisor and anticipate any concerns that may arise with overlapping roles.

C. The physician should tell his neighbor that his new au pair is a patient of his and that he has concerns about her capabilities.

D. The physician should say nothing to anyone.

E. The physician should tell his wife and ask her for advice.

5–6.   Match the landmark legal cases with the quotations.

A. Tarasoff et al. v. The Regents of the University of California
B. Schloendorff v. Society of New York Hospital

5. ____ "The public policy favoring protection of the confidential character of patient-psychotherapist communications must yield to the extent to which disclosure is essential to avert danger to others. The protective privilege ends where the public peril begins."

6. ____ "A surgeon who performs an operation without his patient's consent commits an assault for which he is liable in damages."

7.   Which of the following best expresses the ethical content of the professional responsibility of physicians to their patients?

A. Physicians should fulfill their legal obligations to patients.
B. Physicians should respect the rights of patients.
C. Physicians should responsibly manage organizational resources.
D. Physicians should be honest in all communications with patients.
E. Physicians should fulfill their fiduciary responsibilities to patients.

8–9.   For each of the following scenarios, match the appropriate assessment of the power relationship that exists between the individuals.

A. Equal
B. Unequal

8. ____ Teacher-student

9. ____ Doctor-patient

10–12.   Indicate, on the basis of age, the presumption of decisional capacity for the individuals below.

A. Decisionally capable
B. Decisionally incapable
C. Decisional capacity uncertain

10. ____ Infant

11. ____ 26-year-old

12. ____ 76-year-old

13. A principal investigator discovers that a research assistant on her team has been texting with some of the volunteers on a research protocol. The protocol does not involve texting, because this mode of communication between participants and the research team was not included in the protocol that the institutional review board approved. When the investigator confronted the assistant about this texting, the research assistant responded that the texting has helped with adherence to the research protocol and follow-up; however, he is happy that she raised the issue, because he is somewhat bothered by personal texts he receives from one of the volunteers at all times of the day. Which of the following is the correct next step for the principal investigator to take?
   A. Stop texting immediately, educate the full research staff, explain to the participants how the guidelines prevent further communications by text, and notify the IRB of the situation and action plan.
   B. Text the persistent volunteer, clarifying that the research assistant will not be texting anymore.
   C. Because adherence to the protocol has been effective, maintain the new method of texting and submit an addendum or edit the protocol for the institutional review board.
   D. Because texting has already caused some difficulty, prevent further texting by firing the research assistant for unprofessional conduct.
   E. Ask the research assistant for data supporting improved adherence to the research protocol. If the data prove significant, tell the research assistant that he can keep texting.

14. A gynecologist prescribes an oral contraceptive to a 16-year-old female who is sexually active to prevent pregnancy and to treat dysmenorrhea. Later, her father comes to the clinic, stating that his daughter shared with him that she was placed on this medication and demanding to know why. Which of the following is the most appropriate response and its ethical justification?

   A. Ask that the daughter and father come to the office together for a collective discussion, in order to honor the father's right to be fully informed regarding the medical care of his minor child while also honoring the patient's rights to be involved in this discussion.
   B. Inform the father that patient confidentiality, including state and federal laws, precludes you from answering any questions about his daughter's care as it pertains to this visit.
   C. Fully disclose to the father the specifics of the prescription given and the indications for which it was given (dysmenorrhea and contraception), because she is a minor and it is his parental right to be fully informed regarding her healthcare.

D. Inform her father that she was placed on contraceptives, but the purpose of this prescription was to treat dysmenorrhea, not for contraception. In this way, you can divert his questioning without divulging the sensitive fact that she is sexually active and in need of contraception.

E. In the father's presence, call the patient and obtain her permission to allow her father to read her entire medical record, because you are aware of the ethical duty of the physician to release medical information to a third party at the request of the patient.

15–16. Match the following terms with the description below.

A. Autonomy
B. Beneficence
C. Compassion
D. Expertise
E. Integrity

15. _____ The practice of seeking to support the independent and voluntary decision-making by patients.

16. _____ The practice of seeking to adhere fully to the ideals of the medical profession.

17. A psychiatrist sees a patient in weekly psychotherapy for a year during a period in which the patient is experiencing difficulty with his aging parents and also going through a divorce. Twenty years later, the psychiatrist visits her daughter at college, where her daughter introduces her to her new boyfriend and his father. The psychiatrist recognizes that the boyfriend's father is her patient from years earlier. Which of the following is the psychiatrist's best response to the situation and the ethical justification for her response?

A. Greet the boyfriend and his father without immediately acknowledging knowing the father, because it is the father's choice whether to acknowledge having been in psychotherapy years earlier.

B. Greet the boyfriend and his father and ask the father how things have been going since psychotherapy, because the fact of his being in psychotherapy is bound to come out.

C. Greet the boyfriend and ignore the father, because of their previous psychotherapeutic relationship.

D. Ignore the boyfriend and the father, because of the awkwardness of the social situation and the need to preserve the father's confidentiality.

E. Tell the daughter that she must break up with the boyfriend, because of the need to preserve the father's confidentially.

18. A medical school has a strict policy requiring that all patient billings go through a central billing office. An assistant professor of pediatrics stumbles upon a dermatology clinic that includes, as one of its staff members, a current professor at the pediatrician's medical school. Which of the following is the appropriate course of action for the pediatrician and its ethical justification?

A. Take no action, because of the tradition of professional courtesy.
B. Take no action, because the dermatology professor outranks the assistant professor academically.
C. Take no action, because the economics of the medical school are of no concern to the assistant professor.
D. Notify the chair of pediatrics of the medical school, in order to maintain the integrity of the academic enterprise of the medical school.
E. Set up a pediatric practice on the side like the dermatology professor's, because of the economic advantages that can accrue.

19. A 33-year-old Mexican national who has been living in the United States is employed in an upscale restaurant as a sous chef, earning a modest income in order to take care of himself, his wife, and their two children. He also sends money to México to support his aging parents. Work in the restaurant is very stressful, and he feels tremendous pressure to meet all of his financial obligations. As a result, he visits a community family practice clinic. After he details the stressors in his life, he confides that he has been using an illegal Social Security number in order to get financial and medical benefits. What is the physician permitted to do with this information?

A. Nothing, because the physician is bound by confidentiality laws. The patient can say whatever he wants without the information leaving the office.
B. Nothing, because the physician is bound by confidentiality laws, and the crime does not rise to the level of being reportable.
C. Report this use to the Social Security Administration, the Federal Bureau of Investigation, and Immigration and Customs Enforcement because the patient is committing identity theft and is an undocumented worker.
D. Break the patient's confidentiality and report this use to the local authorities; because the patient is paying the clinic a sliding scale fee, which goes toward the physician's salary, the physician is receiving illegal funds and could be charged as such.
E. Break the patient's confidentiality and report this use to the clinic director and benefits manager. Ask them to close his case, because the clinic can be held culpable for conspiring with and harboring this criminal.

20. An internist prescribes an antihypertensive for an elderly Iraqi man with hypertension. The man is ambivalent about treatment and complies poorly with the medication. His family worries about his condition. The patient's son accompanies him to an appointment and reports that the family has been "sneaking" the antihypertensive into his father's food to ensure that he gets the medication. The patient only speaks Arabic and does not understand what is being said when the son discloses this information. He does not know that he is taking the medication. What should the internist do?

   A. Advise the family to continue.
   B. Increase the dose of the medication in the food.
   C. Report the matter to the police.
   D. Explain to the family the ethical problem with this approach and come up with other methods to improve compliance.
   E. Change the medication to another antihypertensive.

21. A morbidly obese patient is admitted to the hospital for pain control. A surgeon evaluates him and proposes surgery to alleviate his back pain. The patient adamantly refuses surgery because he does not want to abstain from eating in advance of the surgery. Both his primary care physician and his pain specialist want the patient to proceed with the surgery because he has been heavily using pain medication and they are reluctant to prescribe more medications for him. The patient appears to have adequate capacity to refuse the surgery. What ethical principles are in conflict?

   A. Autonomy and beneficence
   B. Autonomy and justice
   C. Fidelity and nonmaleficence
   D. Veracity and beneficence
   E. Veracity and justice

22. A colleague who refers many patients to a physician asks the physician to reschedule her outpatients and see one of his patients for an "emergency" appointment, despite the fact that the patient is not clearly in need of emergency care. The colleague goes on to say his patient is the child of one of the institution's department heads. What should the physician do?

   A. Discuss her overlapping duties (e.g., to him, his patient, and the patient's parent versus the duty to her scheduled patients) with her colleague and arrange for his patient to get appropriate care. No preferential care is indicated.
   B. Report the colleague's unprofessional behavior to his superior and the institution's professional ethics board.

C. See the colleague's patient outside normal clinic hours, at night or on a weekend day, even if this violates the clinic's usual policies.
D. Decline this and all future referrals from the colleague.
E. Reschedule her outpatients and see the colleague's patient as requested.

23–27. Match the legal framework with the relevant established ethical principle.

A. Tarasoff vs. The Regents of the University of California
B. Oregon Death with Dignity Act
C. Griswold vs. Connecticut
D. Superintendent of Belchertown State School and another vs. Joseph Saikewicz
E. Schloendorff vs. Society of New York Hospital

23. ____ Autonomy in medical decision-making is granted to competent adults.

24. ____ Decisions for incompetent patients belong to the legally appointed decision-maker.

25. ____ Patients have a right to reproductive health and right to privacy.

26. ____ Competent adults may request medication to end their lives from their physician.

27. ____ Protected medical record information ends where "public peril begins."

28. A medical school has a strict policy against faculty members receiving stipends from pharmacology companies for presenting lectures. An assistant professor of neurology is at a conference in England when he notices a poster, advertising a lecture by a professor colleague at his medical school touting the effectiveness of a new medication. A pharmacological company sponsors the lecture. Which of the following is the appropriate course of action for the assistant professor and its ethical justification?

A. Take no action, because of the tradition of professional courtesy.
B. Take no action, because the colleague professor outranks the assistant professor academically.
C. Take no action, because the economics of the medical school are of no concern to the assistant professor.
D. Notify the chair of neurology of the medical school, in order to maintain the integrity of the academic enterprise of the medical school.
E. Contact the colleague professor to find out how to get paid for touting the effectiveness of neurological medications in England, because of the economic benefits that can accrue.

29–33. For each of the following descriptions, choose the most appropriate ethics concept. Note that each answer option may be used once, more than once, or not at all.

A. Autonomy
B. Fidelity
C. Nonmaleficence
D. Justice
E. Veracity

29. _____ The duty to behave with honesty and not engage in deception

30. _____ The quality of being faithful to the patient's best interests

31. _____ The capacity to make and enact decisions for oneself

32. _____ The duty to avoid harm

33. _____ The duty to be fair

34–37. Match the legal framework with the correct source.

A. Health Insurance Portability and Accountability Act
B. Tarasoff vs. The Regents of the University of California
C. Oregon Death with Dignity Act
D. Roe vs. Wade

34. _____ Federal statute

35. _____ State statute

36. _____ Federal judicial decision

37. _____ State judicial decision

38–41. For each of the following phrases, match the appropriate ethics term.

A. Altruism
B. Beneficence
C. Compassion
D. Fidelity
E. Respect for persons

38. ____ Promise-keeping

39. ____ Serving others and not oneself

40. ____ Acting to bring about good

41. ____ Recognizing the experience of another person

42. Over several years, a physician diagnosed a wealthy patient with fibromyalgia and directed a successful treatment plan. Before this care, the patient spent roughly 10 years seeing many different physicians with no appropriate diagnosis or treatment for her symptoms. Her quality of life has now improved substantially. At one appointment, she brings a card, noting her appreciation and how the new treatment has positively affected her life. Attached to the card is an envelope with airline tickets and a gift certificate for a weeklong stay at a resort in Hawaii. Which of the following is the most appropriate response and its ethical justification?

  A. Accept the gift graciously – gifts that patients offer to physicians are often an expression of appreciation and gratitude, and it would be insulting and detrimental to the patient-physician relationship to refuse.
  B. Accept the gift graciously – although this gift would likely be inappropriate to accept from a patient with more humble finances, this patient is easily able to afford such a level of expenditure as a gift.
  C. Accept the gift graciously – gifts from patients to physicians often reflect cultural tradition and can enhance the patient-physician relationship.
  D. Decline the gift graciously – provide medication refills to the patient and suggest that she receive care from another physician.
  E. Decline the gift graciously – the gift's value relative to the patient's or the physician's means should not be disproportionately or inappropriately large, and acceptance of such gifts is likely to damage the integrity of the patient-physician relationship.

43–45. Match the following terms with the descriptions below.

  A. Autonomy
  B. Beneficence
  C. Compassion
  D. Confidentiality
  E. Expertise

43. ____ The practice of protecting the personal information of the patient as well as clinical observations about the patient

44. ____ The practice of seeking to bring about the best health outcome for the patient

45. ____ The practice of continuously updating one's medical knowledge and skill

Answers

1. D	16. E	31. A
2. B	17. A	32. C
3. B	18. D	33. D
4. B	19. B	34. A
5. B	20. D	35. C
6. A	21. A	36. D
7. E	22. A	37. B
8. B	23. E	38. D
9. B	24. D	39. A
10. B	25. C	40. B
11. A	26. B	41. E
12. A	27. A	42. E
13. A	28. D	43. D
14. B	29. E	44. B
15. A	30. B	45. E

Recommended Reading

American Medical Association Council on Ethical and Judicial Affairs: Code of Medical Ethics: Current Opinions with Annotations, 2010–2011 edition. Chicago: American Medical Association; 2010.

American Psychoanalytical Association: Ethics Case Book of the American Psychoanalytical Association, edited by Dewarld PA and Clark RW. New York: American Psychoanalytical Association; 2001.

Beauchamp TL, Childress JF. Principles of biomedical ethics. 6th ed. New York: Oxford University Press; 2008.

Boyd KM, Higgs R, Pinching AJ. The new dictionary of medical ethics. London: BMJ Publishing; 1997.

Brems C, Johnson ME, Roberts LW, Warner TD. Healthcare providers' reports of perceived stigma associated with HIV and AIDS in rural and urban communities. J HIV/AIDS Soc Sci. 2010;9(4):356–70.

Coward H, Pinit R, editors. A cross-cultural dialogue on health care ethics. Waterloo: Wilfred Laurier University Press; 1999.

Furrow BR, Greaney TL, Johnson SH, Jost TS, Schwartz RL. Bioethics: Health care law and ethics. 6th ed. St. Paul: Thomson West; 2008.

Geppert CMA, Roberts LW, editors. The book of ethics: expert guidance for professionals who treat addiction. Center City: Hazelden Foundation; 2008.

Grisso T, Appelbaum P. Assessing competence to consent to treatment: A guide for physicians and other health professionals. New York: Oxford University Press; 1998.

Jain S. Understanding physician-pharmaceutical industry interaction – A concise guide. Cambridge: Cambridge University Press; 2007.

Jonsen AR, Siegler M, Winslade WJ. Clinical ethics: A practical approach to ethical decisions in clinical medicine. 7th ed. New York: McGraw-Hill; 2010.

Koenig HG. Spirituality in patient care. 2nd ed. Philadelphia: Templeton Foundation Press; 2007.

Kushe H, Singer P. A companion to bioethics. Oxford: Blackwell; 1998.

Lee E. Working with Asian Americans: A guide for clinicians. New York: Guilford Press; 1997.

Levinson W, Ginsburg S, Hafferty FW, Lucey CR. Understanding medical professionalism. New York: McGraw Hill Lange; 2014.

Lo B. Resolving ethical dilemmas, a guide for clinicians. 3rd ed. Philadelphia: Lippincott Williams & Wilkins; 2005.

Mappes TA, Zembaty JS, editors. Biomedical ethics. 2nd ed. New York: McGraw-Hill; 1986.

Pierce J, Randels G. Contemporary bioethics: A reader with cases. Oxford: Oxford University Press; 2010.

Roberts LW, Dunn LB. Ethical considerations in caring for women with substance use disorders. Obstet Gynecol Clin North Am. 2003;30(3):559–82.

Roberts LW, Dyer A. A concise guide to ethics in mental health care. Washington, DC: American Psychiatric Publishing; 2004.

Sperry L. Dictionary of ethical and legal terms and issues: The essential guide for mental health professionals. London: Routledge; 2007.

The Cross Cultural Health Care Program: Bridging the Gap: A Basic Training for Medical Interpreters. Interpreter's Handbook, Third edition. Seattle: Cross Cultural Health Care Program; 1999.

Williams MA. Practical Ethics in Clinical Neurology. A case-based learning approach. Philadelphia: Wolters Kluwer - Lippincott Williams & Wilkins, 2012.

Veatch RM. The basics of bioethics. 2nd ed. Upper Saddle River: Prentice Hall; 2003.

Chapter 8
Questions on Clinical Issues

Laura Weiss Roberts and Daryn Reicherter

This chapter contains questions from across medical disciplines. The questions are designed to test the learner's understanding of the concepts of professionalism and ethics in medicine as they apply to clinical situations. Correct answers are listed at the end of the section. The learner may refer back to the relevant chapter in Part I for the conceptual framework.

1. A pediatrician working in a neonatal intensive care unit cares for a newborn boy with Down syndrome and a minor degree of esophageal atresia. The boy's parents request that he not receive artificial nutrition or hydration and that he not undergo surgical repair of his esophageal atresia, because they feel their son's life with Down syndrome would not be one worth living. Which of the following is the best course of action for the pediatrician in this case?

    A. Accede to the parents' wishes regarding treatment of their son.
    B. Prepare to start artificial nutrition and hydration of the infant, but avoid consulting a surgeon regarding the medical advisability of surgical correction of the infant's esophageal atresia.
    C. Prepare to start artificial nutrition and hydration of the infant and consult a surgeon regarding the medical advisability of surgical correction of the infant's esophageal atresia.

Contributing authors: Laura Weiss Roberts, M.D., M.A., Daryn Reicherter, M.D., Victor G. Carrion, M.D., Jodi K. Casados, M.D., Cynthia M. A. Geppert, M.D., M.P.H., Ph.D., Michelle Goldsmith, M.D., M.A., Shaili Jain, M.D., Joseph B. Layde, M.D., J.D., Sermsak Lolak, M.D.

L.W. Roberts, M.D., M.A. (✉) • D. Reicherter, M.D.
Department of Psychiatry and Behavioral Sciences, Stanford University School of Medicine, Stanford, CA, USA
e-mail: RobertsL@stanford.edu; dreicherter@stanford.edu

© Springer Science+Business Media New York 2015   125
L.W. Roberts, D. Reicherter (eds.), *Professionalism and Ethics in Medicine*,
DOI 10.1007/978-1-4939-1686-3_8

    D. Administer a lethal dose of potassium chloride to the infant so that his
       parents won't have to see him die slowly.

    E. Personally take the infant to a nearby convent for spiritual care by a
       religious order.

2–3.   Match the following terms with the descriptions below.

    A. Autonomy
    B. Beneficence
    C. Compassion
    D. Expertise
    E. Integrity

    2. ____ The practice of seeking to clarify the patient's preferences for care.

    3. ____ The practice of seeking to recognize and address the sources of
         suffering, discomfort, and burden in the life of the patient.

4–13.   In each of the scenarios below, absolute patient privacy is not maintained.
    For which of the following situations has the privilege of confidentiality
    been formally breached?

    A. Formal breach of confidentiality
    B. Not a formal breach of confidentiality

    4. ____ Members of a healthcare team talking in an unoccupied, closed
         conference room about the details of a patient's care.

    5. ____ Members of a healthcare team talking in the staff cafeteria in the
         hospital about the details of a patient's care.

    6. ____ A member of a healthcare team reporting suspected neglect of the
         patient in a long-term care setting.

    7. ____ A member of a healthcare team reporting suspected neglect by the
         patient of her children.

    8. ____ A member of a healthcare team seeking formal consultation about
         a patient case by a subspecialist at the same hospital, with the
         patient's consent.

    9. ____ A member of a healthcare team talking with the hospital attorney
         about an emerging legal concern in the care of the patient.

10. _____ A member of the healthcare team talking with the patient care ethics committee about an emerging ethical concern in the care of the patient.

11. _____ A member of the healthcare team describing details of a patient's care and identifying information while giving a lecture in the medical school.

12. _____ A quality assurance reviewer evaluating the clinical record for evidence of appropriate standards of care.

13. _____ A quality assurance reviewer discussing with his spouse the details of a patient's care and identifying information in relation to clinical records evaluated at work that day.

14. A hospitalist is treating an elderly woman for systemic infection. The woman is recovering well, but the physician believes it would be safer for her to remain in the hospital for another day or two because of poor support at home. The physician learns that the patient's insurance will not approve the stay unless he "adjusts" some of her medications. He considers changing the dose of her pain and blood pressure medications to satisfy the insurance company's criteria. There is no clear benefit of doing this in a hospital setting, but an additional day or two of admission would clearly benefit the patient's recovery. In this situation, is the physician's decision justifiable?

A. No, this action would constitute deception and falsification of medical records.
B. No, the physician needs to report the woman's family for elder abuse.
C. Yes, the physician's duty is mainly for the patient. The insurance company does not know the patient and makes the decision only for its profit.
D. Yes, the patient is given the best possible treatment, and there is no harmful intention to anyone.
E. Yes, the medications are being adjusted, and there is indication for a longer hospital stay.

15. A medically fragile young woman is listed for solid organ transplant. While awaiting transplant, she becomes increasingly demoralized and depressed. A nurse finds the patient in her room with a pillow over her head, saying, "I cannot go on like this, feeling so sick all the time." A consult is placed for a psychiatric evaluation, and the psychiatrist is asked to attend the next transplant meeting, later that day. At the meeting, without any input from the psychiatrist, the transplant team decides to delist the patient until her depression is treated, understanding that she may die in the interim. The

psychiatrist explains that depression is not a contraindication to transplant, but the team has made its decision. What is the next ethical step for the consulting psychiatrist?

A. Request an emergency meeting of the ethics committee.
B. Treat the patient's depression and hope she gets better soon.
C. Ask the transplant team to reconsider and relist the patient for transplant.
D. Tell the patient that you do not agree with the decision of the transplant team.
E. Tell the patient to go to another hospital to be reevaluated for transplant.

16–18. Match the following terms with the professional duties described below.

A. Autonomy
B. Beneficence
C. Integrity
D. Justice
E. Stewardship

16. ____ An emergency physician provides acute treatment to patients in need irrespective of their background or ability to pay for care.

17. ____ A primary care physician accepts a patient's decision to decline testing for sexually transmitted diseases despite the patient's engaging in high-risk sexual behavior.

18. ____ A transplant surgeon abides by the priority list that is used to determine who receives cadaveric kidneys.

19. When a cardiac interventionist of Indian origin enters a patient's hospital room for a consultation, the patient asks about his ethnic background. Upon learning that he is a "first-generation American," the patient refuses to talk to him further and demands to see someone who is not "an immigrant doctor." The physician is the only person in his specialty who is available in the hospital, and the patient may require an urgent procedure for his condition. What is the most appropriate next step?

A. Politely explain the situation to the patient, explore the patient's concerns, and consult hospital administration or chief medical staff if appropriate.
B. Refer the patient to another hospital.
C. Tell the patient that he has a right to refuse care, but the hospital will not be responsible for the negative outcomes.
D. Call the hospital attorney for the patient's obvious discrimination.
E. Request a psychiatric consultation because the patient clearly lacks capacity to make decisions.

20. A pediatrician is treating a Nigerian adolescent who suffers from "fainting spells." His father does not "believe in doctors" or Western medicine and tells you that his son just needs to get more serious about his academics. The father threatens to remove his son from treatment. What is the best response for the clinician?

   A. Contact child protective services immediately in order to have the child removed from a negligent guardian.
   B. Clarify the father's concerns and provide educational support in order to gain permission for evaluation.
   C. Refer the case to a Nigerian doctor in order to have the treatment clarified.
   D. Send the adolescent to a shelter in an attempt to have him removed from the parent.
   E. Start a medical evaluation secretly with the patient in order to get around the issue of parental consent.

21–24. Match the legal framework to the appropriate clinical case.

   A. HIPAA
   B. Tarasoff vs. The Regents of the University of California
   C. Roe vs. Wade
   D. In Re Karen Quinlan (New Jersey Supreme Court)

   21. _____ A patient with schizophrenia tells his primary care doctor that he intends to kill his landlord because his voices are telling him that the landlord is Satan.

   22. _____ A 19-year-old patient wants to terminate her unwanted pregnancy but is unclear of her legal rights.

   23. _____ A television station calls the hospital to ask about the medical condition of a baseball player injured in a game.

   24. _____ An 80-year-old woman is on life support with limited brain activity after a car accident. Her husband is her health proxy and wishes to discuss the discontinuation of the ventilator.

25–26. Match the following terms with the professional duties described below.

   A. Adherence to the law
   B. Autonomy
   C. Beneficence
   D. Integrity
   E. Justice

25. _____ A pediatrician explains to a parent that there is sufficient concern about a child that a formal report of neglect must be made to the state's Department of Health and Human Services.

26. _____ A surgeon accepts a patient's reasoned decision to decline a recommended operation and to try instead continued intravenous antibiotic treatment for a seriously infected toe.

27. A pediatric patient is orphaned. Her county health insurance has lapsed but will be reinstated when her case is brought to dependency court the following week. In the meantime, the patient will run out of necessary medication. What should the doctor do?

A. Ask the foster parents to pay for the medication out of pocket and hope they receive reimbursement.
B. Provide the medication without telling the patient or the foster parents where it came from.
C. Pay for the medication and receive reimbursement after the insurance is reinstated.
D. Contact the county social worker for input on whom to approach for consent and how to obtain medication in the interim.
E. Tell the patient to wait and that it should be okay to go without medication for a week.

28. A neurology fellow on the consult service is frequently called to the emergency department to evaluate patients with seizure and abnormal movements. One of the attending emergency physicians on the night shift is particularly demanding and verbally abusive to trainee consultants. For example, the physician says that the fellow is taking too long to evaluate the patient, or he characterizes the patients as drunks or people "making up symptoms." The neurology fellow has spoken to her attending physician, but because she is on night float, the neurology attending says not much can be done. What should the neurology fellow do next?

A. Tell the emergency attending physician to "back off."
B. Write up the emergency attending physician for a violation of professionalism.
C. Ignore the emergency attending physician and recognize that not everyone is a team player.
D. Ask one of the neurology attending physicians to accompany the fellow to the emergency department during night float.
E. Consult with the neurology chief resident and training director, and request additional support with how to handle this situation.

29. A 4-year-old Native American child presents with her mother for a standard well-child check. The history and physical exam reveals that she is healthy and demonstrates development that is appropriate for her age. It is time for her standard childhood immunizations. Her mother states that she does not want her child to have any of these immunizations, because she is concerned about the risks of Western medicines. She states that she prefers to use natural, Native American herbs to keep her child healthy and she does not feel that it is necessary or safe for her child to have the immunizations. *Streptococcus pneumoniae* infections are prevalent at the reservation where they live, making the need for vaccination more pressing. Which of the following is the most appropriate response and its ethical justification?

    A. Call child protective services.
    B. Educate the patient's mother on the medical justification for the immunizations.
    C. Administer the vaccinations regardless of the mother's objection, because the physician's ethical duty is to act in the best interests of the patient.
    D. Discontinue treating the child, because of disagreement with the mother's desire to use alternative forms of medicine.
    E. Assure the mother that the vaccinations are 100 % safe and effective.

30–31. Match the following terms with the descriptions below.

    A. Privacy
    B. Confidentiality
    C. Secrecy

    30. ____ Legal privilege granted to patients that requires physicians to keep patient information private unless compelled to make a disclosure or the patient gives consent.

    31. ____ State or quality of keeping things concealed or hidden.

32. An infectious disease specialist at a busy community hospital is routinely consulted by a colleague from internal medicine. He notices a concerning trend in the prescribing pattern of his colleague. She starts antibiotics very quickly on her patients, before receiving full test results of samples and before she knows the sensitivity of the microorganisms involved. Moreover, the antibiotics she uses are very new and the specialist has concerns about the unknown side effects of these newer medications over tried and tested older medications. Also, the new antibiotics are expensive and it is hard to justify the cost to the patient. Which of the following is the most appropriate course of action for the infectious disease specialist?

   A. Do not accept any new consults from this colleague.

   B. Do not cancel her orders; she has been a good source of referrals and the service needs to show it is productive.

   C. Cancel her orders and prescribe older antibiotics once the sensitivities are known and the microorganisms identified.

   D. Offer to do an in service, to her and her team, on the benefits of conservative approaches to the prescribing of antibiotics.

   E. Report the colleague to the licensing board.

33. An ophthalmologist elected to a hospital administrative committee seeks to identify highly effective generic medications for inclusion on the hospital pharmacy formulary. Which of following ethical terms best describes the ophthalmologist's action?

   A. Autonomy
   B. Beneficence
   C. Integrity
   D. Justice
   E. Stewardship

34. A cardiologist has treated a patient for many years. The patient's symptoms recently deteriorated, so the cardiologist wants him evaluated for possible cardiac transplant. The cardiologist, however, is also a member of the transplant selection committee. When the patient's case is presented, other committee members express concerns about the patient's candidacy because of his poor support system and possible pain medication abuse. The cardiologist truly believes that the patient would do well after the transplant and on many occasions has given the patient the impression that he would have no problem being on the transplant list. What is the appropriate action for the cardiologist in this situation?

   A. Refer the patient for independent psychosocial evaluation, and excuse himself from the role of selection committee member when the committee discusses this patient.

   B. Refer the patient for independent psychosocial evaluation, but maintain the role of committee member, because he knows the patient well and already fully discloses his roles.

   C. Discuss the patient with the other committee members before the meeting to convey his optimism for the patient's candidacy.

   D. Refer the patient to another transplant center to avoid conflict of interest.

   E. Refer the patient to a new cardiologist, but maintain the role of committee member when the committee discusses this patient.

35. A primary care physician refers a patient to a gastroenterologist for consultation. Upon reviewing the patient's medical records and history, the gastroenterologist finds evidence that the primary care physician provided treatment to the patient that was not evidence based and would be consider substandard. What is the most appropriate first step?

   A. Call the primary care physician and gently discuss the concerns, to increase understanding of the situation.
   B. Do nothing. The primary care physician has a full license, and it is not the gastroenterologist's role to judge the primary care physician's clinical competence.
   C. Call the state board of medicine and report the primary care physician's malpractice.
   D. Encourage the patient to switch primary care physicians immediately and report the primary care physician to the state board of medicine.
   E. Tell other doctors to avoid referring any patients to this primary care physician.

36–40. Match the most relevant statement regarding decisional capacity to the individual patient scenarios below.

   A. Presumed decisionally capable.
   B. Presumed decisionally capable, but may require evaluation for capacity for consent.
   C. Presumed decisionally incapable.
   D. Presumed decisionally incapable, but may require evaluation for capacity for consent.

   36. _____ A 57-year-old diabetic man develops an infected toe and accepts recommended IV antibiotics.

   37. _____ A 57-year-old diabetic man develops an infected toe and declines recommended IV antibiotics.

   38. _____ A 6-year-old healthy boy develops an infected toe and accepts recommended IV antibiotics.

   39. _____ A 14-year-old healthy boy develops an infected toe and accepts recommended IV antibiotics.

   40. _____ A 14-year-old healthy boy develops an infected toe and declines recommended IV antibiotics.

41. A patient tells her friend, "The doctor said that I shouldn't take antibiotics for a virus." Which of the following elements of capacity for informed consent is demonstrated in this statement by the patient?

A. Evidence of capacity to appreciate the nature of the decision
B. Evidence of capacity to reason through the decision
C. Evidence of capacity to understand information relevant to the decision
D. Evidence of capacity to make a voluntary decision

42–49. The American Board of Internal Medicine Professionalism Project has identified several behaviors illustrative of professional and unprofessional conduct. For each of the behaviors noted below, indicate whether the behavior is indicative of professional conduct, unprofessional conduct, or not relevant to professional conduct.

A. Professional conduct
B. Unprofessional conduct
C. Not relevant to professional conduct

42. ____ "Lack of effort toward self-improvement and adaptability."

43. ____ "Lack of sensitivity to the needs, feelings, and wishes of the healthcare team."

44. ____ "Conscientious effort to exceed ordinary expectations and to make a commitment to lifelong learning."

45. ____ "Recognition of the possibility of conflict of interest and avoidance of relationships that allow personal gain to supersede the best interest of the patient."

46. ____ "Demonstrates arrogance."

47. ____ "Is overly critical/verbally abusive during times of stress."

48. ____ "Needs continual reminders about fulfilling responsibilities to patients and to other healthcare providers."

49. ____ "Discussion of details of patients' situations in public."

50–54. For each of the following pairs, indicate whether the procedures/interventions are listed in the correct order or incorrect order with respect to the need for an increasingly rigorous standard for capacity for informed consent.

A. Correct order
B. Incorrect order

50. ____ Blood draw for cholesterol check, blood draw for genetic test.

51. ____ Intravenous antibiotics, oral antibiotics.

52. ____ Oral medication, depot injection medication.

53. ____ Overnight sleep study for clinical purpose, overnight sleep study for clinical research purpose.

54. ____ Emergency hospitalization of patient, demand by patient for discharge against medical advice.

55. A patient from a remote area with a non-ST elevation myocardial infarction is transferred to a major urban academic medical center for urgent cardiac catheterization. All the members of the cardiology team caring for him are from other countries. The patient begrudgingly allows the team to examine him but repeatedly makes racist and demeaning statements about their ethnicity. Which of the following is the most appropriate response to the patient's behavior and its ethical justification?

A. Accept the patient's behavior and arrange for him to be transferred to a cardiology team with only American-born physicians and trainees.
B. Accept the patient's behavior, but make it clear that he is a racist and the staff does not like his attitude.
C. Do not accept the patient's behavior; tell the patient that hospital policy does not allow patients to demean staff and he will be reported to management.
D. Do not accept the patient's behavior; calmly and professionally tell the patient that such remarks will not be tolerated and he must treat all members of the healthcare team with respect.
E. Do not accept the patient's behavior; tell the patient that if he does not apologize to the team for his comments, he will not receive the catheterization.

Answers

1. C	20. B	39. D
2. A	21. B	40. D
3. C	22. C	41. C
4. B	23. A	42. B
5. A	24. D	43. B
6. B	25. A	44. A
7. B	26. B	45. A
8. B	27. D	46. B
9. B	28. E	47. B
10. B	29. B	48. B
11. A	30. B	49. B
12. B	31. C	50. A
13. A	32. D	51. B
14. A	33. E	52. B
15. A	34. A	53. B
16. D	35. A	54. A
17. A	36. A	55. D
18. D	37. B	
19. A	38. C	

Recommended Reading

American Medical Association Council on Ethical and Judicial Affairs: Code of Medical Ethics: Current Opinions with Annotations, 2010–2011 edition. Chicago: American Medical Association; 2010.

Beauchamp TL, Childress JF. Principles of biomedical ethics. 6th ed. New York: Oxford University Press; 2008.

Boyd KM, Higgs R, Pinching AJ. The new dictionary of medical ethics. London: BMJ Publishing; 1997.

Coverdale JH, Balon R, Roberts LW. Teaching sexual history-taking: a systematic review of educational programs. Acad Med. 2011;86:1590–95.

Coward H, Pinit R, editors. A cross-cultural dialogue on health care ethics. Waterloo: Wilfred Laurier University Press; 1999.

Furrow BR, Greaney TL, Johnson SH, Jost TS, Schwartz RL. Bioethics: Health care law and ethics. 6th ed. St. Paul: Thomson West; 2008.

Grisso T, Appelbaum P. Assessing competence to consent to treatment: A guide for physicians and other health professionals. New York: Oxford University Press; 1998.

Jain S. Understanding physician-pharmaceutical industry interaction – A concise guide. Cambridge: Cambridge University Press; 2007.

Jonsen AR, Veatch RM, Walters L. Source book in bioethics: A documentary history. Washington, DC: Georgetown University Press; 1998.

Jonsen AR, Siegler M, Winslade WJ. Clinical ethics: A practical approach to ethical decisions in clinical medicine. 7th ed. New York: McGraw-Hill; 2010.

Koenig HG. Spirituality in patient care. 2nd ed. Philadelphia: Templeton Foundation Press; 2007.

Kushe H, Singer P. A companion to bioethics. Oxford: Blackwell; 1998.

Kushner TK, Thomasma DC. Ward ethics dilemmas for medical students and doctors in training. Cambridge: Cambridge University Press; 2001.

Lee E. Working with Asian Americans: A guide for clinicians. New York: Guilford Press; 1997.

Lo B. Resolving ethical dilemmas, a guide for clinicians. 3rd ed. Philadelphia: Lippincott Williams & Wilkins; 2005.

Mappes TA, Zembaty JS, editors. Biomedical ethics. 2nd ed. New York: McGraw-Hill; 1986.

Pierce J, Randels G. Contemporary bioethics: A reader with cases. Oxford: Oxford University Press; 2010.

Roberts LW. Informed consent and the capacity for voluntarism. Am J Psychiatry. 2002;159:705–12.

Roberts LW, Battaglia J, Smithpeter M, Epstein RS. An office on main street: health care dilemmas in small communities. Hastings Cent Rep. 1999;29(4):28–37.

Roberts LW, Dyer A. A concise guide to ethics in mental health care. Washington, DC: American Psychiatric Publishing; 2004.

Roberts LW, Geppert CM, Warner TD, Green Hammond K, Lamberton L. Bioethics principles, informed consent, and ethical care for special populations: curricular needs expressed by men and women physicians-in-training. Psychosomatics. 2005;46(5):440–50.

Roberts LW, Hoop JG. Professionalism and ethics – Q&A self-study guide for mental health professionals. Washington, DC: American Psychiatric Press; 2008.

Roberts LW, Roberts BB, Warner TD, Solomon Z, Hardee JT, McCarty T. Internal medicine, psychiatry, and emergency medicine residents' views of assisted death practices. Arch Intern Med. 1997;157:1603–9.

Spellecy R, Roberts LW. Developing your ethics skills. In: Roberts LW, Hilty DM editors. Handbook of career development in academic psychiatry and behavioral sciences. Arlington: American Psychiatric Press; 2006. p. 133–46.

Sperry L. Dictionary of ethical and legal terms and issues: The essential guide for mental health professionals. London: Routledge; 2007.

The Cross Cultural Health Care Program: Bridging the Gap: A Basic Training for Medical Interpreters. Interpreter's Handbook, Third edition. Seattle: Cross Cultural Health Care Program; 1999.

Veatch RM. The basics of bioethics. 2nd ed. Upper Saddle River: Prentice Hall; 2003.

Chapter 9
Questions on Research and Education

Laura Weiss Roberts and Daryn Reicherter

This chapter contains questions from across medical disciplines. The questions are designed to test the learner's understanding of the concepts of professionalism and ethics in medicine as they apply to research and training. Correct answers are listed at the end of the section. The learner may refer back to the relevant chapter in Part I for the conceptual framework.

1. A third-year medical student is invited to shadow an attending physician preceptor on an intensive care unit. The student notices that one of the second-year medical students has been admitted to the unit. The third-year student is sincerely concerned about the well-being of her second-year classmate and wonders what the student-patient's condition might be. Which of the following is her best course of action?
   A. Ask the attending physician about the student-patient's medical condition and the reason for admission.
   B. Go to the student-patient directly to express emotional support and learn what is happening.
   C. Obtain the student-patient's electronic medical record and review it.
   D. Post an announcement on the second- and third-year medical student class' social networking site.
   E. Refrain from inquiring about the student-patient and maintain confidentiality.

Contributing authors: Laura Weiss Roberts, M.D., M.A., Daryn Reicherter, M.D., Michelle Goldsmith, M.D., M.A., Joseph B. Layde, M.D., J.D., Sermsak Lolak, M.D., Teresita A. McCarty, M.D., Christine Moutier, M.D.

L.W. Roberts, M.D., M.A. (✉) • D. Reicherter, M.D.
Department of Psychiatry and Behavioral Sciences,
Stanford University School of Medicine, Stanford, CA, USA
e-mail: RobertsL@stanford.edu

© Springer Science+Business Media New York 2015
L.W. Roberts, D. Reicherter (eds.), *Professionalism and Ethics in Medicine*,
DOI 10.1007/978-1-4939-1686-3_9

2.   During a rotation on an inpatient medicine service, a resident tells a peer
      that he has taken "just a few" opiate pills out of the medication-dispensing
      machine. What should the peer do?

      A. Nothing, because the event was not witnessed.
      B. Nothing, but watch for future impairment or misconduct.
      C. Encourage the resident to get mental health help and report the
         disclosure to the Residency Training Director.
      D. Speak to a neighbor who happens to be an attorney about the situation.
      E. Report the disclosure to the State Medical Board.

3–5. For the scenarios below, choose the most appropriate term for the resident's
      decisions and actions.

      A. Professional behavior
      B. Unprofessional behavior

      3. _____ A resident forgets to order a routine laboratory test in the care of
               a hospitalized patient and informs his attending the next day.

      4. _____ A resident forgets to order a routine laboratory test in the care of a
               hospitalized inpatient and informs his attending the next day that the
               "lab messed up."

      5. _____ A resident forgets to order a routine laboratory test in the care of
               an outpatient and calls the laboratory to add the test "stat" even
               though it will incur additional cost for the patient's insurance.

6–7. A young girl with advanced cancer is enrolled in a research study with a
      randomized, controlled design that compares an innovative treatment with
      usual clinical care for her illness. The intent of the protocol has been care-
      fully explained to the parents, and they express clear understanding of the
      factual information related to the study. Match the scenarios below with the
      ethical term or phrase used to characterize a concern in informed consent
      for research.

      A. Insufficient voluntariness
      B. Misinformation
      C. Therapeutic misconception

      6. _____ That evening, the mother confides to her sister, "We just know that
               the doctors will give her the experimental medicine – they are such
               good doctors and they seem to love her almost as much as we do!"

      7. _____ That evening, the mother confides to her sister, "We just did not
               know what else to do – our insurance ran out and getting her into
               this study was the only way we could get her any treatment at all!"

8. A resident informs a patient that she is a physician-in-training and will be supervised by a senior attending in providing the patient's clinical care. Which one of the following terms matches the professional duty the resident is demonstrating?

   A. Adherence to the law
   B. Autonomy
   C. Beneficence
   D. Integrity
   E. Justice

9. A chief resident learns that a male resident has flirted with several female residents, made unwanted advances after being told to stop, and in one instance waited outside a resident's apartment in his car, followed her in, and trapped her in a closet. They are all willing to speak with the chief resident and even provide her with evidence from letters, a card, and a videotape but refuse to call the police or speak with the Office of Prevention of Sexual Harassment for fear of reprisal. What action should the chief resident take?

   A. Nothing, because the female residents are not willing to come forward to anyone but the chief resident.
   B. The chief resident should consult with her supervisor, training director, and the Office of Prevention of Sexual Harassment.
   C. The chief resident should inform the other female residents that if they do not report the incidents, the male resident may only be disciplined via informal mechanisms, if at all.
   D. The chief resident could provide information to the other female residents about protection against reprisal that would likely be afforded them under the Whistle-Blower Act.
   E. The chief resident should call the police and present the evidence of stalking.

10–14. Indicate whether the activity described meets the criteria for human research according to the US Department of Health and Human Services regulations.

   A. Does not meet criteria for human research
   B. Does meet criteria for human research

   10. ____ Careful and systematic review of public websites for relevant health information of celebrity patients cared for at the hospital where a researcher works.

   11. ____ Careful and systematic review of medical records for relevant health information of celebrity patients cared for at the hospital where a researcher works.

12. _____ Careful and systematic review of laboratory results for community residents who live near the hospital where a researcher works.

13. _____ Careful and systematic review of published obituaries for relevant
health information for community residents who live near the hospital where a researcher works.

14. _____ Careful and systematic review of pathology reports of patients
who have died at a hospital where a researcher works.

15–18. Indicate whether the following statements are correct or incorrect.

A. Correct
B. Incorrect

15. _____ Research protocols involving greater risk entail more careful
informed consent.

16. _____ Confidentiality is protected equally in human research and in clinical care.

17. _____ Institutional Review Boards are solely responsible for the oversight of risks and safety in human research protocols.

18. _____ All human research occurring in an academic medical center
should be approved or formally deemed exempt from review by
its own or an affiliated Institutional Review Board.

19. All third-year medical students complete out-of-class assignments in a sim-
ulated electronic medical record as part of a final exam. They receive written and oral instructions prohibiting the use of reference materials. All final
examination exercises are designed to be the work of individuals. The clinical instructor typically follows student progress electronically during the
exam, and it becomes clear that two students are working together. The
instructor meets with the students individually and asks for an explanation.
One student explains that he was so worried about the medical record por-
tion of the test that he asked his fellow student for assistance. He adds that
he found it very helpful to work with his friend and that they both learned a
lot. The second student states emphatically that they did not collaborate on
the examination and then breaks down and admits that they did work
together. Both students say it did not occur to them that working together

was unacceptable and they think other students must work together too. Choose the most appropriate term for the students' decisions and actions.

    A. Professional behavior
    B. Unprofessional behavior

20. A volunteer in a double-blinded, placebo-controlled, randomized clinical trial for a chemotherapeutic medication tells the physician that she thinks she is getting the placebo because the IV bag leaked and the contents were without odor. Other volunteers during infusion have mentioned how bad the IV fluid smells. The volunteer is upset and wants to be switched to the other arm of the trial. What should the physician do?

    A. Switch the volunteer to the other arm of the trial.
    B. Remove the volunteer from the study and thank her for her participation. Provide follow-up care with approval from the Institutional Review Board.
    C. Explain to the volunteer the importance of having participants in both the placebo and medication arms of the study and her need to remain in the arm to which she was randomly assigned.
    D. Explain to the volunteer that there is no way of knowing which arm of the study she is in because the study is double-blinded and even the physician does not know the answer. She should remain in her assigned condition.
    E. Tell the volunteer that the medication is odorless and there is no way of knowing what she is getting.

21. A pediatrics training director reading through the personal statements of applicants for first-year positions in the residency program notices that two are very similar. Both applicants tell first-person stories about coming to love pediatrics after treating a 3-year-old girl whose mother suffers from multiple sclerosis. Several key phrases are the same. Which of the following is the best course of action for the training director and its ethical justification?

    A. Report the appearance of plagiarism to the Association of Pediatric Program Directors to maintain the integrity of the application process.
    B. Ignore the similar stories, because personal statements in applications are unimportant.
    C. Ignore the appearance of plagiarism, because it is too difficult to pursue plagiarists.
    D. Invite the two applicants to interview on the same day in order to confront the plagiarism.
    E. Invite both applicants to interview because of the heartwarming nature of their personal statements.

22. A psychiatrist at a medical school is in charge of the student mental health service. He also takes call on the consultation-liaison service in the university hospital once a year. A medical student whom the psychiatrist has been treating for depression is rotating through the consultation-liaison service when the psychiatrist is the attending physician. Which of the following is the best course of action for the professor and its ethical justification?

   A. Keep the medical student off the rotation to preserve the confidentiality of her treatment for depression.
   B. Arrange for the medical student to have a different attending for her rotation, because of the dual nature of the treating and supervisory relationship the psychiatrist would have with her.
   C. Fail the medical student for the rotation, because of what the psychiatrist has learned while treating her.
   D. Inform the dean's office that the medical student should not take a psychiatry rotation, because she is in treatment for depression.
   E. Give the student a grade of honors in the rotation, because of her courage in facing her depression.

23. An MD/PHD student has developed a research proposal and needs a clinical site for data collection. A physician in charge of a clinic on her academic medical campus offers her access to data in exchange for authorship credit. The student is not sure if this contribution warrants authorship but fears losing the opportunity. What should the student do?

   A. Ask the clinic physician if she can be first author and he can be second.
   B. Contact her dissertation advisor for guidance.
   C. Inform the clinic physician that he can be an author because it is a student project.
   D. Report to the office of academic affairs that the clinic physician harassed her.
   E. Agree on the condition that the clinic physician would give her authorship on his next paper.

24. The chairman of an internal medicine department hears from several residents that one of the attending physicians has been spending a lot of time socially with a resident. Other residents report that the resident involved has spoken while intoxicated at a party about the infatuation he and the attending doctor have for each other. Which of the following is the best course of action for the chairman and the ethical justification for it?

   A. Fire the attending physician, because of the appearance of favoritism that the relationship could cause.

B. Fire the resident, because the possible relationship with a supervisor is inappropriate.
C. Ignore the reports, because they are hearsay.
D. Ignore the situation because it does not represent an ethical dilemma.
E. Counsel the attending physician and the resident separately about the inappropriateness of relationships between supervisors and trainees because of their inequality at work.

25–28. Match the scenarios below with the ethical term or phrase used to characterize a concern in research integrity.

A. Conflict of interest
B. Conflict of role
C. Honest mistake
D. Research error
E. Research misconduct

25. ____ Working under an exceptionally tight deadline, a researcher makes an incorrect calculation in analyzing his data for an upcoming scientific presentation.

26. ____ Discovering that one of six experiments was not conducted, a researcher documents that the experiment was done, accurately imputing the data from the five other experiments.

27. ____ Using conventional scientific methods that are later found to be inherently flawed, a researcher draws a conclusion from his data that turns out to be incorrect.

28. ____ Trying to meet a recruitment deadline for a clinical trial, a researcher intentionally ignores a relevant aspect of a potential volunteer's clinical history.

29–35. Conscious and unconscious biases introduce the possibility of prejudicial attitudes shaping the views and decisions of physicians when interacting with patients, patient families, and colleagues. For each of the following scenarios, indicate whether there is evidence of conscious and unconscious bias that may influence the situation.

A. Evidence of conscious and unconscious bias is apparent.
B. Evidence of conscious and unconscious bias is not apparent.

29. ____ A patient says to a female surgical resident, "A woman surgeon! Crazy. Don't you want to have a family?"

30. _____ A patient says to a male OB-GYN resident, "How can a man do this job well?"

31. _____ A patient says to a female resident, "You are so young! How can you be a doctor? You must be smart."

32. _____ A patient says to a female resident, "I am glad you are my doctor – I don't trust anyone over 40!"

33. _____ A patient says to a male medical student, "Do you have any tattoos? I have a lot, but I wish I hadn't gotten them on my hands – can't get a job that way."

34. _____ A patient says to a female resident, "Hey, howya doing, Doc?"

35. _____ A patient says to a male resident, "Hey, howya doing, Doc?"

36. A medical student asks a patient for permission to perform a thoracentesis. It will be the first time that the medical student has done a thoracentesis, although she has watched others perform the procedure several times and a very experienced resident will supervise her. The patient asks her how many times she has performed a thoracentesis. Before she can respond, the resident says, in an exaggerated, bored manner, "You don't even want to know how many times she's done this." Which of the following is the medical student's most appropriate response to the resident's statement?

A. Address the issue immediately and openly by saying, "The resident is teasing me. This is the first time I've done this procedure."
B. After completing the procedure, report the resident to the program director for unprofessional conduct.
C. Because the resident did not lie and the patient was reassured, adopt the resident's approach and use it again in similar situations.
D. Leave the patient room immediately and report the situation to the hospital attorney.
E. Smile and nod in front of the patient but afterward consult a faculty member about how to handle the resident in the future.

37–38. A medical student has designed a project in which he will ask his fellow students to respond to a survey assessing attitudes toward their curriculum and will correlate their perspectives with their background characteristics and personal health habits. He will employ confidentiality safeguards. For the scenarios below, choose the most appropriate term for the student's decisions and actions.

A. Honest mistake
B. Research error

37. ____ The student carefully reviews the human subjects regulations and sees that his project meets criteria for being "exempt" from review, so he conducts the project without contacting the Institutional Review Board.

38. ____ The student speaks with his faculty advisor, who has carefully reviewed the human subjects regulations and sees that his project meets criteria for being "exempt" from institutional. She tells him that he does not need further approval, and he conducts the project without contacting the Institutional Review Board.

39–41. A medical student notices that the chief resident on her rotation neglects to do thorough physical examinations on unattractive patients but, with great fanfare, thoroughly examines attractive patients. She wonders if she has imagined this bias, because she believes that all of the patients receive excellent care. Near the end of the rotation, she mentions this pattern to her intern, who responds, "Oh, yeah. You got that right! We always have to go back and double-check everything. You should see the chief with the VIPs! It's even worse! And I don't think he realizes it!" For the scenarios below, choose the most appropriate term for the student's decisions and actions.

A. Professional behavior
B. Unprofessional behavior

39. ____ The student does not discuss this observation with others again but documents it in her feedback form at the end of the rotation.

40. ____ The student chats informally with her intern everyday about the pattern for the remainder of the rotation but decides not to mention it in her feedback form for fear of retaliation.

41. ____ The student decides not to mention the pattern in her feedback form at the end of the rotation but tells the two students rotating next on the ward about her observation and encourages them to "double-check everything, just in case."

42–44. For each of the following descriptions, choose the most appropriate ethical principle.

A. Altruism
B. Beneficence
C. Compassion
D. Justice
E. Nonmaleficence

42. ____ A researcher offers a study volunteer "comfort medications" to help with the transition to a difficult phase of a clinical protocol.

43. ____ A researcher ensures that each arm of a clinical trial offers treatment equivalent to the "standard of care" for an illness.

44. ____ A study volunteer understands that it is unlikely she will benefit from participating in a cancer clinical trial but hopes that it will help "the next person" who suffers similarly with the disease she has.

45. A pathology professor peer-reviews for several medical journals. While reviewing a manuscript submitted to him anonymously, the pathologist finds that the author is claiming credit for developing a new tissue stain that the reviewer had developed a year earlier. Which of the following is the appropriate action for the reviewer and the ethical justification for it?

A. Review the manuscript and make no comment about the reviewer's own development of the stain, because that is the gracious thing to do.
B. Include in the manuscript review the fact that the reviewer had developed the stain earlier, in order to maintain the integrity of the scientific process.
C. Demand that the journal disclose who authored the paper, in order to defend the reviewer's intellectual property.
D. Refuse to review any more manuscripts for the journal, because the journal accepts manuscripts from thieves.
E. Review the manuscript with an extremely critical eye toward its writing style in order to prevent the paper from reaching publication, so that the theft of intellectual property is punished.

46. A fellow in surgical oncology completes a research project and writes most of a manuscript outlining the research. She receives minimal assistance from the professor who is her advisor on the research, but when the time comes to submit the paper for publication, the professor insists on being named first author. Which of the following is the resident's best course of action and its ethical justification?

A. Submit the paper for publication with the professor named as first author, because rank trumps effort.
B. Do not submit the paper for publication, because of the need to maintain the integrity of the publication process.
C. Discuss the situation with the surgical oncology program director to ensure that the resident receives first author credit and her supervisor does not take improper credit for intellectual work.

D. Name the professor as first author but post a blog entry decrying the unfairness of the academic system.
E. Withdraw from the fellowship because of the professor's interference with intellectual rights.

47. While reviewing the curriculum vitae of a fellowship candidate, a training director notes a gap in time of one year when the individual was not in work or school. During the interview, the director asks her what she did during this time. She replies that she was travelling abroad and remarks on countries visited and memorable occasions. A physician who wrote one of her letters of reference happens to be a colleague of the director from residency. The director contacts him regarding the candidate, and the physician shares confidentially that she was ill during that time period, took a leave of absence, and then returned to medical school. Prior to this inconsistency, the director had considered her an outstanding candidate. What should the director do?

A. Discuss the inconsistency with the candidate's other references.
B. Discuss the inconsistency with the candidate without revealing the source.
C. Do not discuss the inconsistency because it does not make any difference.
D. Do not discuss the inconsistency with the candidate because it does not represent a pattern of behavior.
E. Do not discuss the inconsistency with the candidate, but note the issue in the evaluation of her application to share with the ranking committee.

48–50. For the scenarios below, choose the most appropriate description.

A. Professional boundary crossing
B. Professional boundary violation
C. Neither

48. ____ Resident begins dating a patient.

49. ____ Second-year medical student begins dating another second-year medical student.

50. ____ An attending physician begins dating another attending physician.

51. A patient who has struggled to get a job asks the resident physician in the primary care clinic to sign a form to continue his disability benefits. The resident is not fully convinced that the patient cannot work, but if the resident refuses to sign the form, the patient may risk losing money and becoming unable to afford medications that are essential for his health. The resident speaks with the attending physician, who encourages the resident to make his own decision on the report. What ethical principles are in conflict as the resident physician arrives at an ethical decision?

   A. Beneficence and confidentiality
   B. Beneficence and nonmaleficence
   C. Fidelity and justice
   D. Justice and veracity
   E. Nonmaleficence and veracity

52–55. For each of the following pairs, indicate whether the protocols are listed in the correct order or incorrect order, with respect to the need for an increasingly rigorous standard for review by the Institutional Review Board.

   A. Correct order – Protocol 1 poses a more favorable risk to benefit ratio than protocol 2.
   B. Incorrect order – Protocol 2 poses a more favorable risk to benefit ration than protocol 1.

   52. ____ Protocol 1: Web-based anonymous survey of attitudes toward fast food by resident physicians at a preventive health conference conducted by a nearby hospital.

      Protocol 2: Paper-based confidential survey of attitudes toward fast food by resident physicians conducted by their supervising attending at their training hospital.

   53. ____ Protocol 1: Project to study lean body weight and exercise patterns of employees of a large local employer.

      Protocol 2: Project to study lean body weight and exercise patterns of recently incarcerated parolees of a large local prison.

   54. ____ Protocol 1: Project to study genetic vulnerabilities in healthy elders residing in the community.

      Protocol 2: Project to study genetic vulnerabilities in chronically ill elders residing in a long-term care facility.

55. _____ Protocol 1: Project that randomizes healthy people to receive placebos vs. vitamins while withholding all other medications.

Protocol 2: Project that randomizes arthritis patients to receive placebos vs. vitamins while withholding all other medications.

Answers

1. E	20. B	39. A
2. C	21. A	40. B
3. A	22. B	41. B
4. B	23. B	42. C
5. B	24. E	43. E
6. C	25. D	44. A
7. A	26. E	45. B
8. D	27. C	46. C
9. B	28. E	47. B
10. A	29. A	48. B
11. B	30. A	49. C
12. B	31. A	50. C
13. A	32. A	51. B
14. A	33. A	52. A
15. A	34. B	53. A
16. B	35. B	54. A
17. B	36. A	55. A
18. A	37. B	
19. B	38. A	

Recommended Reading

American Medical Association Council on Ethical and Judicial Affairs: Code of Medical Ethics: Current Opinions with Annotations, 2010–2011 edition. Chicago: American Medical Association; 2010.

Beauchamp TL, Childress JF. Principles of biomedical ethics. 6th ed. New York: Oxford University Press; 2008.

Boyd KM, Higgs R, Pinching AJ. The new dictionary of medical ethics. London: BMJ Publishing; 1997.

Brody BA. The ethics of biomedical research: An international perspective. New York: Oxford University Press; 1998.

Cassem N, Jeste DV, Roberts LW, et al. Research involving individuals with questionable capacity to consent: ethical issues and practical considerations for institutional review boards (IRBs). Expert Panel Report to the National Institutes of Health (NIH), February 1998.

Dunn LB, Misra S. Research ethics issues in geriatric psychiatry. Psychiat Clin North Am. 2009;32:395–411.

Hoop JG, Roberts LW, Green Hammond K. Genetic testing of stored biological samples: views of 570 U.S. workers. Genet Test Mol Biomarkers. 2009;13(3):331–7.

Hilty DM, Leamon MH, Roberts LW. Approaching research, evaluation, and continuous quality improvement projects. In: Roberts LW, Hilty DM, editors. Handbook of career development in academic psychiatry and behavioral sciences. Arlington: American Psychiatric Press; 2006. p. 273–84.

Hulley SB, Cummings SR, Browner WS, Grady DG, Newman TB. Designing clinical research. Philadelphia: Lippincott Williams & Wilkins; 2006.

Jain S. Understanding physician-pharmaceutical industry interaction – A concise guide. Cambridge: Cambridge University Press; 2007.

Jonsen AR, Veatch RM, Walters L. Source book in bioethics: A documentary history. Washington, DC: Georgetown University Press; 1998.

Jonsen AR, Siegler M, Winslade WJ. Clinical ethics: A practical approach to ethical decisions in clinical medicine. 7th ed. New York: McGraw-Hill; 2010.

Katz J. Experimentation with human beings. New York: Russell Sage Foundation; 1972.

Kushe H, Singer P. A companion to bioethics. Oxford: Blackwell; 1998.

Kushner TK, Thomasma DC. Ward ethics dilemmas for medical students and doctors in training. Cambridge: Cambridge University Press; 2001.

Lehrmann J, Hoop JG, Green Hammond K, Roberts LW. Medical students' affirmation of ethics education. Acad Psychiatry. 2009;33(6):470–77.

Machin D, Campbell MJ. The design of studies for medical research. Wiley: Chichester; 2005.

Mappes TA, Zembaty JS, editors. Biomedical ethics. 2nd ed. New York: McGraw-Hill; 1986.

Miles SH, Lane LW, Bickel J, Walker RW, Cassel CK. Medical ethics education: coming of age. Acad Med. 1989;64:705–14.

Pierce J, Randels G. Contemporary bioethics: A reader with cases. Oxford: Oxford University Press; 2010.

Roberts LW, Dyer A. A concise guide to ethics in mental health care. Washington, DC: American Psychiatric Publishing; 2004.

Roberts LW, Hoop JG. Professionalism and ethics – Q&A self-study guide for mental health professionals. Washington, DC: American Psychiatric Press; 2008.

Rothstein WG. American medical schools and the practice of medicine: A history. Oxford: Oxford University Press; 1987.

Spece Jr RG, Shimm DS, Buchanan AE. Conflicts of interest in clinical practice and research. New York: Oxford University Press; 1996.

Roberts LW, Geppert CM, Connor R, Nguyen K, Warner TD. An invitation for medical educators to focus on ethical and policy issues in research and scholarly practice. Acad Med. 2001;76(9):876–85.

Roberts LW, Geppert CM, McCarty T, Obenshain SS. Evaluating medical students skills in obtaining informed consent for HIV testing. J Gen Intern Med. 2003;18:112–19.

Roberts LW, Geppert CM, Warner TD, Green Hammond K, Lamberton L. Bioethics principles, informed consent, and ethical care for special populations: curricular needs expressed by men and women physicians-in-training. Psychosomatics. 2005;46(5):440–50.

Roberts LW, Mines J, Voss C, Koinis CN, Mitchell SM, Obenshain S, McCarty T. Assessing medical students' competence in obtaining informed consent. Am J Surg. 1999;178:351–4.

Roberts LW, Roberts BB, Warner TD, Solomon Z, Hardee JT, McCarty T. Internal medicine, psychiatry, and emergency medicine residents' views of assisted death practices. Arch Intern Med. 1997;157:1603–9.

Roberts LW, Warner TD, Dunn LB, Brody JL, Green Hammond K, Roberts BB. Shaping medical students' attitudes toward ethically important aspects of clinical research: results of a randomized, controlled educational intervention. Ethics Behav. 2007;17(1):19–50.

Roberts LW, Warner TD, Green HK. Coexisting commitments to ethics and human research: a preliminary study of the perspectives of 83 medical students. Am J Bioethics. 2005;5(6):W1–7.

Roberts LW, Warner TD, Green Hammond K, Brody JL, Kaminsky A, Roberts BB. Teaching medical students to discern ethical problems in human clinical research studies. Acad Med. 2005;80(10):925–30.

Veatch RM. The basics of bioethics. 2nd ed. Upper Saddle River: Prentice Hall; 2003.

Index

© Springer Science+Business Media New York 2015
L.W. Roberts, D. Reicherter (eds.), *Professionalism and Ethics in Medicine*,
DOI 10.1007/978-1-4939-1686-3